MIRACLE

James D Richardson

MIRACLE

A TRUE STORY

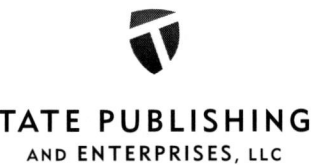

TATE PUBLISHING
AND ENTERPRISES, LLC

Miracle: The James D. Richardson Story
Copyright © 2012 by James D Richardson All rights reserved.

No part of this publication may be reproduced, stored in a retrieval system or transmitted in any way by any means, electronic, mechanical, photocopy, recording or otherwise without the prior permission of the author except as provided by USA copyright law.

The opinions expressed by the author are not necessarily those of Tate Publishing, LLC.

This book is designed to provide accurate and authoritative information with regard to the subject matter covered. This information is given with the understanding that neither the author nor Tate Publishing, LLC is engaged in rendering legal, professional advice. Since the details of your situation are fact dependent, you should additionally seek the services of a competent professional.

Published by Tate Publishing & Enterprises, LLC
127 E. Trade Center Terrace | Mustang, Oklahoma 73064 USA
1.888.361.9473 | www.tatepublishing.com

Tate Publishing is committed to excellence in the publishing industry. The company reflects the philosophy established by the founders, based on Psalm 68:11,
"The Lord gave the word and great was the company of those who published it."

Book design copyright © 2012 by Tate Publishing, LLC. All rights reserved.
Cover design by Joel Uber
Interior design by Lucia Kroeger Renz

Published in the United States of America

ISBN: 978-1-62024-407-4
Biography & Autobiography / Medical
12.06.19

ACKNOWLEDGMENTS

I have so many people that I need to thank. I have personally thanked all of these people, but I would like to thank them this way as well! My wife, Leslie (I will always be there for you), and Mom and Dad Dopke, Momma FOG (thank you for all of those great dinners!), my mom and dad, thank you for all your support. I love you all so much! My "hero" and my biggest angel, Dr. L. Schwartz. Dr. S. Schwartz, the best oncology doctor in the world. Dr. Apostolou, the best surgeon in the world; Dr. Hart, the best radiation doctor in the world; Dr. Belen and Dr. Kaplan, the best pulmonary doctors in the world. Karen, Melanie, and Penny are all angels to me! There are many doctors behind the scenes I want to thank as well. You know who you are, and my heart goes out to you!

I want to thank everyone at DMC Huron Valley Hospital!

I want to thank all of my family for their support, especially Jerry and Ruth, Mark and Tara, and Kristie.

I want so say special thanks to my friends, Tom and Jill, Tommy and AJ, Randy and Judy, and Andrea.

There are so many other people to thank that it would be another book in itself!

My most important thank you is to God! Thank you for giving me another chance. I won't let you down!

TABLE OF CONTENTS

INTRODUCTION............................9

THE FIRST SIGNS OF SYMPTOMS.......... 11

WAS I STUPID............................ 19

COURAGE TO MOVE ON................... 31

THE NEW DOC........................... 37

THE MIRACLE........................... 73

THE SURGERY........................... 103

GETTING READY FOR CHEMO AGAIN.... 135

THE CANCER SURVIVORS' PARTY 195

STAYING FOCUSED...................... 199

THE CANCER CAME BACK 207

MAKING IT BACK TO WORK............. 217

CONTACT INFORMATION 221

INTRODUCTION

This story is about my fight with stage-four inoperable lung cancer and how I survived.

    I am writing this book in the hope to inspire people. I want to give hope back to someone who lost it. This is my story, and it is a true story. If you have a serious illness and need inspiration to go on in life or a need to restore your faith in God, please read my story. It is a true miracle that I survived. I hope you will enjoy it as much as I have enjoyed writing it. God bless you all!

    Sincerely,
    James D. Richardson

THE FIRST SIGNS OF SYMPTOMS

This story you're about to read has drastically changed my life forever. It's a true story about courage, fear, faith, hope, love, and inspiration. Life was great for me. But when you're not expecting it... Just when you think, it won't happen to you...

It was spring 2009. It had been such a long winter. All my brothers and I could talk about was getting out and playing golf. Last fall we both had spent a ridiculous amount of money on new "top of the line" clubs thinking it would improve our games. I looked like a pro PGA player out there. At least for me it didn't help at all. As far as I am concerned it was a waste of hard-earned money. My brother came up with this saying to make us both feel better about it, "At least we look good." I shrugged my shoulders and went along with it at the time. We had planned our first trip for the year. We were going to Jerry's house to stay for a long weekend and to play some of his local golf courses. I was looking forward to seeing Jerry and Ruth. We live far apart and don't get to see each other often. I was on the phone with Jerry just before the trip. I was telling him about how I had developed some back pain in my upper back and my hands. He was asking me if I wanted to cancel the trip. I said, "Not a chance."

I said, "I know my job can be pretty physical at times, but something is not right. I just don't feel right."

I figured that I just pulled another muscle in my back again, and I left it at that. As the golf trip was approaching, my knees and ankles began to swell and ache a little. I started to feel very fatigued every day. I was thinking about what my doctor meant when he said, "Welcome to the forties." It's hell getting old, isn't it? Whatever way you want to look at it. I wanted answers. I was telling my wife just before the trip how badly I was hurting and how tired I felt all the time. She was saying to me to please go back to the doctors. I said that I would when I got back from the golf trip.

As the weekend approached, I was feeling pretty rough, but I wanted to go up north and play golf. It was our first time out for the season. So I decided to go play golf with my brothers anyway. My brother-in-law was going, and he asked if he could drive this time. I thought that would be great, since I was feeling so rough. He came over to pick me up, and we were on our way up north.

I was looking forward to the trip. I was excited to see Jerry and Ruth. On the way up there, we talked about the family and the issues that were going on. It helped me take my mind off of my problems (the expensive golf clubs I recently purchased and being sick) and made them seem little after that car ride. Three hours later, we arrived. We were ready to tear it up and have a good time. We were all glad to be together again. It doesn't happen often.

We all said our hellos and unloaded the car. We loaded up Jerry's large Buick with all of our golf clubs and headed to the golf course. It's called Tustin Trails. It's a great nine-hole course. We all really enjoy playing this course. It's well-kept and groomed. We got to the golf course and stopped up front at the bag drop. Jerry let us all out there, and he went to go park the car.

We walked in the clubhouse and paid our green fees. Jerry was talking with the owner, so I decided to go out and sit in a cart and get everything ready to go. As I sat in the cart waiting for my brother, my ankles and knees started to swell up and ache a little more. I just couldn't believe this was happening to me. I had some Tylenol in my golf bag. I got some out and took a couple to help with the aches and pains. My brothers finally came out, and we started to play.

The first hole was rough. Getting a six on a par four? Hey, what could I say, we were out having a good time. The second hole was a par three. It's a hole you have to hit over the water. There is something psychological about hitting the ball over water. Alternatively, maybe the golf balls are attracted to water. My brothers and I did not do so well. They also had that mental issue about hitting over the water. I really do not know what is so funny about watching a guy or gal tee up a ball and hit it in the water. I laugh every time. Usually my side hurts afterward. After my brother-in-law hits his into the water he slams his club down onto the ground and yells out "son of a gun" and "damn it" every time. It's pretty damn funny!

"A couple of eights," they said. Just to rub it in a little I said, "Puddin' (that's his nickname) what did you get again?"

"You know damn well what," he said.

He would slam his club in the bag. We laughed with him, or at him I guess. I really don't remember why we call him Puddin'. It just stuck one day. They smiled, and I wrote the scores down. My knees were hurting so badly that I could barely stand to finish the nine holes. My hands were aching badly. It began to rain very lightly. It was not a hard rain but enough to get you wet. I was standing there in the rain, waiting for my next shot. I was looking at my grip when I noticed a little change in my fingernails and tips. It was as if my fingertips were getting wider. I was staring at them thinking, What the hell is going on? With the swelling issue and the rain, I had no focus. It was definitely affecting the game. We finished up and headed home.

We got back to my brother Jerry's place, and we began to talk about my health issues. My brother was surprised to see me this way because I have always taken pretty good care of myself. Although I smoked back when I was younger, I still worked out and ran when I could. When I quit smoking, I gave it up for good. Do you want to know how I quit? That's good because I am going to tell you anyway. I was driving home from work thinking about my kids and what would happen to them if they lost their dad to cancer.

What would they do without their dad? I rolled the window down and threw them out the window. That's right. I tossed the whole pack and the lighter. I quit cold turkey and never looked back. When I got a craving to smoke I did something to take my mind off of it like think of my children. After all they were a gift from God himself. I did it because it was best for me. After all, I deserved to be free from their chains, and so did my kids. You should too if you smoke. My brother and I talked about the first time we smoked. We both got sick as hell. That alone should have been the first clue not to do it. I told him when I got home that I would go back to the doc's office to find out what was going on. In the meantime, I needed to put my ankles and knees on some ice to help with the swelling. My ankles had swelled up to twice their normal size. Whatever was going on definitely had my full attention.

For the evening, we hung around the house and ordered some pizza and played poker for the rest of the night. While I was lying in bed I was thinking about my little girls and how special they are to me. I thought of a time when we went to pick up their bunk beds. They wanted to share a room together pretty badly. My oldest was seven years old and the little one was three years at the time. When we left to shop for them we told them they could pick them out. We went from furniture store to furniture store searching for the right ones. As we would walk through the store they would jump from bed to bed laughing and having a good time.

I would say, "That's enough girls," and the salesmen would say, "It's all right, dad, they are having fun." The looks on their faces and the giggling and laughing was what was great. Finally they picked out the ones they wanted. It was this loft style set with a desk at one end. On the way home with it my oldest expressed how she wanted the top to sleep in. I quickly agreed. We got home and they begged me to assemble the beds right away. After many "please daddys" I agreed and went to work on it. Many hours later, and I mean many, it was finally finished. I woke the girls from the couch where they fell asleep waiting for me and put them in their new beds.

They both were awake and wanted to play on it. I insisted they go to sleep and tucked them in for the night. The next morning my oldest was up early and had come into my room to wake me up. I was sound a sleep. She made a few attempts to shake my leg to wake me. She gave up and climbed onto my bed and then sat on me. She grabbed my eye lashes, one with each hand, and pulled them both open, yelling, "Wake up daddy! Wake up!"

I said, "I am awake. Now let go of my eyelashes please."

She let go and began to giggle and said, "I tried pushing you to wake you first."

I could not help but laugh. It was the way she said it I guess. She was so adorable.

I said, "What's so important?"

"Thank you for the bunk beds, Dad! They are awesome!"

I smiled at her and said in a very sleepy voice, "You are very welcome. Where is your little sister?"

She said, "She is still asleep."

I looked over at the clock and it was 6:02 am. I said, "I guess we are up for the day, huh?"

She giggled some more.

I said, "I'll go make breakfast for us while you go play."

She agreed and went back to her room. While I was cooking scrambled eggs my youngest came running up to me yelling "Daddy" and hugged my legs.

She said, "Thank you, Dad," and ran back into her room. She was so precious. God, I miss those moments. I felt so blessed to have had them.

Look at me now. I thought, "Where did that time go?" and went to sleep.

Morning had come, and my knees and ankles were doing okay. The swelling had gone down at least. The pain was mild as well. We decided to go out for breakfast before we went to play the next course. After we ate, we were headed to McGuire's Resort to play golf. Before we left the parking lot at the restaurant, it started to rain again. Either way, I said to the group that I was all right with the rain. I came to play golf, rain or shine. The rest of the group decided to go play as well.

We arrived at the course and loaded up our carts. I was doing everything I could to focus on the game and try to enjoy myself. My vacations are so few and far between. It was about the third hole when the swelling started again. By the fourth hole, I was hurting so badly that I just sat in the cart until they finished playing.

"Something is seriously wrong with me," I said to my family.

They were asking me if I was able to make it. I said I wouldn't be able to play anymore. I was telling Ruth how bad my hands ached and that I could barely hold the club with the swelling.

The morning came, and my brother-in-law and I loaded up the car. We said our good-byes and headed home. It was a quiet ride home. We got home, and I thanked my brother-in-law for driving. I looked over at him and said I would drive next time. He smiled and said, "Not a chance."

We unloaded my gear, and he headed home. (He just doesn't like my Mustang convertible; it makes him have motion sickness.) It was Saturday evening, and I was talking to my wife, Leslie, about what was going on with my health.

We went downstairs to the family room to watch our favorite soap, General Hospital. All the soaps were recorded, of course, on the DVR. We had a couple of weeks to catch up on, so we made a night of it. We watched General Hospital and talked about the golf trip a little. The swelling came back right along with the pain. It did not take much for me to call the family doctor this time.

WAS I STUPID…

It was Monday morning, and I got up to call and make another appointment with the family doctor. Within a few days, I was in the doctor's office, telling him about the problem. I was telling him about my knees, ankles, and hands swelling and hurting, and the back pain I had was still there from a previous visit to him. I was feeling very fatigued and weak. I also explained the change taking place with my fingertips.

He stood there looking at me and said, "I have decided to give you a bone density exam and take more blood for testing."

I said, "Doctor, I'm still having that pain in my back."

He said, "Those take time to heal."

I said, "How about an X-ray?"

He still would not take an X-ray of my back. After the exam was over, he wrote me a prescription for a steroid step-down pack and told me to take some Aleve to help with the joint pain. He felt I had some form of arthritis. He referred me to go see his doctor friend that was an arthritis specialist.

"It's all I can do for you now," he said. "I'll talk to you soon." He walked out of the exam room.

So I got up and was going to the checkout area. I was standing in line listening to the office women complaining about overbooking his patients and making them wait for long periods of time. I stood there thinking how glad that I was not to be the only one feeling this way.

When it was my turn to check out, I decided to express my feelings on the waiting and said, "I will not wait any longer than a half an hour from this day forward. I understand that there are emergencies. I have no problem with that. I do have a problem when a greedy doctor is overbooking patients and pushing people through like cattle on a farm. How could a doctor help his patients if he doesn't listen to them? He is in and out of the exam room so fast. He couldn't have been in there no longer than a minute."

She agreed that it was ridiculous.

I said to have a good day, and I left for work. By the way, I work the second shift, 3:00 to 11:30 p.m. I sat in my car, trying to get enough courage just to go to another doctor. For some reason, I hate changing doctors. Maybe it was because I was lazy and did not want to fill out any more paperwork.

That evening, it started all over again. The swelling and the pain were ridiculous. I was thinking, How in the hell am I going to get through the night? It was one step at a time. I got home and took a shower and climbed in bed. Leslie asked how I was doing. I said to her that I was doing okay and that I was just tired. I left it at that. I did not want her to worry about me because she had the full plate as it was with her work and family.

When I got up the next morning, I called to schedule an appointment to see one of the doctors at the arthritis office. I explained to them who referred me and the symptoms I had. I said to the women, "My ankles and knees are swelling up. My hands and wrists have been swelling as well. My back is hurting in the upper and lower areas. I need to see the arthritis doctor right away, please."

They got me in right away within a few days. This is one reason why I do not like switching doctors. The first doctor I had seen didn't think he could help because he was in the knee-replacement area of medicine. So he referred me to another female doctor in the same office that was an expert in the field of arthritis. Don'tcha just love the medical racket!

So I had to reschedule another appointment and wait another week. Yes, it was BS! For you babies who are reading, that means "bad stuff." I had expressed my feelings about the confusion to the woman at the reception desk.

I said to her, "One would think when you call and schedule an appointment and explain what's wrong with you that they would give you the right doctor."

She just stared at me with a stupid look on her face. She treated me as if I were one of those people on the stranger danger lists, if they even have one of those lists. It was how I felt at the time. Anyway, I just left.

I had a tough time getting through the week at work. The pain was getting worse. I was not getting anywhere with my family doctor. The steroids were not working at all. I was hoping this woman doctor had the answers to my problems.

Finally, it was the appointment day. I got in there to meet the new doctor. I was explaining to her how I had back, knee, ankle, and hand pain and swelling. I pointed out that my fingertips were changing. I told her about how my upper- and lower-back pain had been around for a while now.

I also explained to her that I have UC (ulcerative colitis). As she gave me an exam, she started to explain to me that she didn't think I had UC but that I had Crohn's disease instead. She felt the swelling was a form of a side effect from the Crohn's disease. She told me that my gastrointestinal doctor misdiagnosed me. She seemed upset with the guy and had no doubt in her mind that I definitely had Crohn's disease.

"How could he have missed this?" she said.

I was thinking to myself, How can she tell all of this without doing a colonoscopy? Either she's really good or off her rocker.

As I sat there listening to her, I felt that she seemed confident and well educated. She went on about arthritis and was telling me that I had seronegative arthritis. That's a side effect of the Crohn's disease. I sat there and processed the information for a moment. I thought maybe she was right. You're supposed to trust what your doctor says, right? Maybe I did have Crohn's after all. I needed to know what was wrong with me. She started to tell me about a drug called Humira and that she thought it would take care of the issue.

She explained how it was self-injected, or I could come there every other week to get shots. I said that I would have to give that one some thought. I don't want to sound like a 230-pound baby, but I was not excited to inject myself with these big needles.

She said, "In the meantime, I would like to have some X-rays done here at my office."

I said okay, and she left to set it up. I thought, Finally, I will get X-rays of my back.

After a few minutes, the X-ray technician came and took me back to have the X-rays done. She took X-rays of my hands, knees, and feet.

I asked the technician, "What about my back?"

She said those were the entire X-rays the doctor requested. I thought to myself, Why not my back?

She took me back to my exam room, and I got dressed. I waited for the doctor to return. A couple of minutes later, she came back with some info on the Humira drug. I asked her again about my back. She went on about how it probably was a pulled muscle, and she felt the Humira would take care of it and that it was part of the arthritis. I decided to trust this doctor after all. What did I know? I was just a janitor.

It was the second week in June, and I was willing to try anything at this point. I was hurting so badly. So I decided to try it. The arthritis doctor had ordered a Crohn's/arthritis Humira kit. I decided to go with the self-injections. She told me that in order for me to take this medication, I had to pass a couple of tests. I had to go get more blood work done and go get a TB test done at my family doctor's office. She sent me on my way.

School was out, and it was time for summer cleanup. By the way, just in case you were wondering what janitors do at the school over the summer, the whole school gets cleaned from top to bottom. All the walking was killing me. At this point, I was taking more breaks than my supervisor. I continued to tough it out one step at a time. I had scheduled an appointment to get the TB test done and blood work done at the same time. When I arrived at Doctor Overbooking's office, I was not surprised to see the lobby full.

I waited twenty-five minutes before I was called back to the exam room. I then waited another twenty-five minutes for Doctor Overbooking to come in with another college trainee of his. I said to the trainee, "Could you excuse us, please?"

He looked at the doctor for an okay.

The doctor said, "It's okay. I will be out in a second."

The trainee left the room. I said to the doctor that I had enough players in the game right now and to recap what's going on here. I asked him if he had spoken with Dr. Arthritis yet.

He said, "I did speak with her, and she feels you have arthritis. She did mention the new drug she wanted to put you on. I didn't know about it, and I'll have to research it."

I said, "Here, take mine."

I gave him the information the arthritis doctor gave me. I said, "Look, Doc, I am giving you all of my trust on this. I do hope you research it. By the looks of the lobby, you will not have time."

He just smiled.

I smiled back. I think I made my point without too much damage. After all, I was not out to embarrass him.

He said the nurse would be back in a minute to give me the TB shot and walked out. The nurse came into the room smiling and said good morning. I said good morning back. She just kept smiling and gave me the shot on the arm.

She said, "Don't forget to come back in two days."

I said, "Okay. Have a good day."

I was walking to check out when I heard the nurses talking about what I said to the doctor about the overbooking. I guess someone overheard. Oops!

I went back in a few days to have the TB results read. The lobby was still full, and I still had to wait twenty-five minutes. I thought that was long enough to wait, so I walked up to the receptionist desk. I said, "Hi! Are you a nurse?"

She said, "Yes, I am."

I said, "Well." I handed her my paper to be signed for the TB test. "Will you look at my arm and sign off, please."

She looked at me for a moment and went to say something. I just cut her off with, "I have been sitting out here for over twenty-five minutes to have a TB test read. Now if you would, please sign this, so I can be on my way to work."

She took the paper and signed it.

I said, "If the doctor is angry at you, just give him my number and blame me for it." I pointed out that my number was on my chart file on the cover. I said thank you to her and walked out. I was good to go.

I took the results back to the arthritis doctor's office. I asked if the blood work came back yet. The receptionist said not yet. So I left for work. The arthritis doctor's office called in a few days with the results and said I was all set to go. I waited for the Crohn's Humira injection kit to arrive in the mail. Humira is a very expensive medication. I was told that it cost $700 an injection. The kit contained six injections. Thank God I have medical insurance, I was thinking at the time.

About another week had passed, and I went back for a follow-up appointment with Dr. Overbooking. I pointed my fingers out to the doctor about the clubbing. The doctor was looking at my fingers. He stated that they were clubbing and said this happened to people that have arthritis. He felt sure of himself that that was what I had. He had asked me what the arthritis doctor had to say. So I explained to him everything and about the Humira drug again.

I explained that I was waiting for it to come in the mail. I told him about all the X-rays she did, and she thought the back pain was possible arthritis and that the Humira should take care of it. He stood there with a blank look on his face for a moment. As he stood there looking at my chart, he said to me that everything seemed fine to him.

"The bone-density test results came back and looked fine," he said. "I feel we're on the right path here. Let's see what the Humira drug does for you. Go over to the

DMC office for more blood work. Have a good day." He walked out.

Do you ever get the feeling doctors are not listening to you? I just left to check out. He clearly was not paying attention. I don't think he remembered that I just had blood work done a couple of weeks ago.

July was here, and I was on vacation. I took the whole week off to be with my family. I was divorced and had gotten remarried back in 2005 to a beautiful woman inside and out! I have two girls from my previous marriage as I said earlier. I was excited to see my girls (my babies!). I don't get to see them often but every other weekend. My oldest daughter just started her senior year of high school. I was so proud of her! My youngest was fourteen years old.

It was a great week other than my health. Every day was a struggle getting around, but I did my best not to complain. I tried very hard to do chores around the house, mowing and trimming the grass, picking up dead tree limbs and help with the cleaning inside. "Domestic duties" we all love. My mustang was a convertible and required hand washing to keep the top from being beat to death from the automatic car wash. My girls helped me wash it. The Humira kit had come at this time, and I gave myself the injections. I started to explain to my kids what was going on and that I would keep them posted. We spent a lot of time hanging out at the house.

We talked about the old days at our previous home. They reminded me of the ride in the Barbie Jeep my youngest had gotten for her fourth birthday and how much fun they had in it. She expressed how excited she was when she had seen the large wrapped box. My youngest daughter loves adventure. We knew it would be the perfect gift for her. At the time she wanted to be an archeologist when she got older. My oldest daughter reminded my youngest that when she opened it she remembered her being overwhelmed with excitement and could not open the box fast enough.

We all spent a few hours assembling the Jeep, placing stickers everywhere and laughing because I could not put it together fast enough. I must have heard "Are you done yet, Dad?" twenty times or so. After I finished the interior they smiled as they climbed into the Jeep and were checking out its entire features. After I installed the charged battery and closed the hood my oldest daughter walked around the Jeep making sure they had everything they could think of for their first expedition. They had put water bottles in the cargo net and a couple of their toys to bury. I explained to them to always wear their seatbelts.

My oldest daughter laughed at me as she mimicked me saying in a deep voice, "No exceptions, girls. No seatbelts, no Jeep!" We all laughed together. What can I say? I was worried about there safety.

Afterward, she said that as they explored the back yard in the Jeep it felt like they were in a different part of the world. Their imaginations went crazy.

They dug holes with their little plastic shovels and would bury certain items to be dug up later. The dogs would chase them as they drove around. They would act as if there were wild animals after them. They remembered having so much fun. We laughed a little about the steep hill in the backyard. The Jeep would not climb the steep hill at all. They would get so frustrated with that.

They would yell, "Dad, come and push us!" That particular night after the battery was dead I added some small screws to the rear wheels for traction. It helped a lot; it made it to the top anyway. It was great to reminisce with them. I miss them so much. I hated the rules of divorce. Only being to see them every other weekend was BS! Those babies being taken away from me tore a hole in me wider then the Grand Canyon. I will never get that time back, those moments. After all, I did not have them not to be with them. At this point I cherished every minute I had left. We watched the fireworks from the bridge this year. They were spectacular. The girls enjoyed them a lot. We spent time with our neighbors and good friends and had a few campfires. The girls and I set up tents in the backyard for them to sleep in when their cousins were over. They had a blast giggling and laughing into the night.

The next week, I went to the arthritis doctor again. I told her I was not doing any better. I still had the back pain and the swelling issues. She told me to give the Humira some time to work, at least six weeks. I was so miserable. I was thinking to myself, I don't have six weeks.

Dr. Arthritis prescribed me some Tylenol 3 to take to help with the pain.

So I went on my way. I did my best that I could at work and at home. I tried to stay focused on the positive things in life. I watched movies in our family room. I spent time with my dogs in the backyard, throwing the ball. I loved my wife every second I could when she was not working. She is so loved and appreciated. I need her like a human needs a heart to live.

COURAGE TO MOVE ON

It was August now, and the six weeks had passed. The Humira was not working at all. I decided to quit taking the Humira. I felt in my heart that this was not a good medication to take for me. I went back to see the arthritis doctor to see what else we could do. I told her about all the pain I was in. I said that it was time to try something stronger than Tylenol. She gave me a pain medication prescription to try. I told here the swelling was getting worse as well.

I said to her that I was flat-out miserable. I remember I was practically begging for help. She talked me into trying Humira for a couple more shots. So I did what you should never do. I went against my heart and followed her direction and hoped that it would work. I was having a very difficult time getting in and out of the car. At work, I struggled and could barely finish every day. I was so weak that I thought I was dying. I tried to spend as much time as I could relaxing around the house.

In September Leslie and I decided it was time to get away for a long weekend and go and hang out with friends. We were invited to a friend's motel on Lake Huron. There were eight couples getting together for a fun, action-packed weekend. Tom and Jill were explaining all the fun things to do up there. For me it was just about hanging out and relaxing. I needed it. We packed up the Mustang and headed out.

I quickly stopped at the end of the driveway and said, "I forgot something!"

"What?" Leslie asked.

I pulled the latches to the top and put the top down.

"There," I said. "Now we are ready," and I slowly backed out, staring at Leslie.

Leslie smiled and said, "You have issues, convertible boy."

I said, "I know I do," and smiled at her. "If you have a convertible, you have to use it, right?"

The weather was beautiful, and the trees began to change color. As I drove, Leslie and I talked about all the possibilities that could be wrong with me. There were so many. We agreed once we got there not to talk about it amongst the friends until we had answers. I smiled at her and held her hand for a while. It was so fun to be with her. She is so loved! When we got there the sun was shining and some of the friends were out on the jet skis jumping waves and racing each other. The rest of the pack was hanging out at the beach. We waved to them as we unloaded the car. The cooler had all of our favorite things in it, rum, coke, some beer, potato chips, pretzels, and animal crackers. They're cholesterol free... (Kids, do not drink at all, it's so bad for you, and for you outlaws and rebels that do, do not drive!) Let me be a role model for you—Adults, drink responsibly!

We switched into our bathing suits and walked down to the beach to be with them. It was so relaxing there. I decided to walk up the shoreline a little with my feet splashing in the water. The water was so cold. It felt nice because my feet and ankles hurt. I was so grateful to be alive. I was having a hard time with this illness situation. My focus on life was all messed up as well. My trust for my doctors was gone. It did not take long for my ankles to swell up a little so I headed back. When I returned they had started a bonfire in the pit. I could hear the wood crackling as I approached.

The burning lumber smelled wonderful. Leslie brought a portable radio for everyone to listen to. I pulled up a chair on top of a sand dune and stared way out at the water, watching large ships pass by and thinking how blessed I was to have great friends and to be loved. I listened to friends talk about their lives and how great things were for them. I was happy for them all. After a few hours of hanging out at the beach we went into town for a late dinner. Afterward, we headed back to the bonfire pit to hang out some more and have a couple drinks.

What made this night interesting was a large group of girls from a softball team were staying at the motel that weekend as well. They had started a bonfire farther down the beach. As the night progressed we pulled out the rum bottle and had a few beers to drink. It helped take my mind off of my problems. Leslie and I laughed with our friends as we heard stories from them. A couple of hours later the girls from the softball team decided to go skinny dipping. Tom pointed over my shoulder when he noticed a couple of them walking out into the water.

The first thing I heard from other friends was, "Holy smokes! There is a God after all!" The radio was turned down.

Leslie quickly turned to look and said, "Those are some brave girls." That water was ice cold. I couldn't believe this was happening before our very eyes.

Someone yelled, "Are they filming a movie here?" We all laughed out loud and looked for cameras just in case. After all, none of us had seen anything like that before. It was like something you would see in a Hollywood film. We all stared at them as more of the girls from the team joined in.

One of the guys yelled, "Could someone turn a light on please!" We all laughed some more. For a few minutes it was really quiet in our group as another friend had said, "I should come up here more often." We all started laughing and went about our business. The girls from the softball team had kept to themselves and we had a great weekend relaxing with friends. On the way home we took our time and laughed about the craziness that happened. It was so nice to get away even if it was only for a few days. Sorry, no pictures.

After a few weeks, I went back to Dr. Overbooking's again for a follow-up. Nothing changed here at this time. He still passed me on to other colleagues and would not listen to me at all. You want to talk about something frustrating as a patient? Nobody likes to be passed on and treated like they don't matter when they're seriously ill. My back, knees, ankles and, by this time, my hands were completely hurting, and my fingers looked fully clubbed.

I was miserable and going nowhere with these two doctors. It was time to move on. I went on to work and got through the night the best I could. When I got home, I talked with my wife about finding a new doctor to go to. Leslie was so frustrated. Maybe you can relate to this. You know when your child or a loved one is ill and your heart goes out to them. You feel so sorry for them. You want to help them the best you can, but you can't because you're not God or Jesus. This would be my beautiful bride Leslie. She recommended that I see her doctor. The next day I called and set up an appointment with him. As I stated earlier, I hated the thought of switching doctors.

It took a couple of weeks to get in to see him. At this point, I had quit taking the Humira. It was not helping at all. I should have followed my heart weeks earlier. It was the night before the appointment with the new doc. I was lying in bed, just absolutely pissed at myself for not having the courage to move on earlier. I was mad at myself because I trusted those two doctors, and it almost cost me my life! To this day, I feel they led me on to get my insurance money.

I was stupid enough to be led on by them. There are a lot of doctors out there that will take advantage of you and tell you things you do not need. Since I switched doctors, I have found that not all doctors are like this, just some! If I can say anything to help another person, it is to find the courage in you to move on sooner than I. It just may save your life! Don't waste seven months of your life being miserable like I did. Now I feel if you listen to your heart, you are usually right!

THE NEW DOC

It was appointment day with the new doctor on November 17, 2009, and I was looking forward to meeting him. My wife had so many great things to say about him. When I got there, it was nice to find it was not overbooked. I still had to fill out more paperwork. I waited for a short time and was called to go back to the exam room. After a few minutes, the new doctor came in.

"Hello," he said, "my name is Dr. Schwartz. It's very nice to meet you finally. I have heard so many great things about you from Leslie. All of us here are excited to meet you finally."

I shook his hand. Right away, I liked how confident he was. There was something about him that made me feel comfortable. He asked me what was going on. I started telling him my situation and what had happened with the other two doctors and what I had been through.

I was telling him about the pain I could not seem to get rid of in my upper back. I went on about my fingers changing and the swelling I had in my hands, knees, ankles, and feet. So right away, he wanted to take an X-ray of my back. I thought, "Finally someone willing to take an x-ray." I instantly loved this guy. I had a smile on my face if you could only imagine. He went to set it up. After a few minutes, the X-ray technician came to get me. After we were done, she sent me back to my exam room. I got dressed and waited for the doctor to return. I figured he would say, "Man, that's a nasty pulled muscle." However, when he came back, he looked stressed and frustrated.

He said, "I don't even know how to say this to you."

I said, "Just shoot me straight, Doc. I can handle it."

"Well," he said, "it doesn't look good! Doc held up the x-ray to the light so I could try and understand what he was saying. He pointed things out as he spoke. You have a very large tumor in your right lung. It is so large that it looks like the tumor has grown through your lung. This is where the pain is coming from in your back."

I was just blown away by the news. I sat there for a minute to process the news. I looked at the doctor in the eyes and said I would be the one to tell my wife. Doc and Leslie had known each other for a long time, since my wife had been young. They used to work together. Regardless of their relationship, I wanted to be the one to tell her the news.

I said to him, "What's the next step?"

Dr. Schwartz said, "Let's get a bronchoscopy done. Where do you guys live exactly?"

I said, "Over by the Huron Valley DMC hospital."

Doc said, "Perfect. We can set up a CAT scan there. I know the perfect doctor to handle the bronchoscopy."

I said, "Okay."

"I know a couple of really good surgeons that can help you as well. You should talk with one of them to see what they think. In the meantime, I will talk with the hospital about the CAT scan. Let's do this right away before you meet the surgeon or anyone else. You should schedule an appointment with Dr. Belen to meet him."

He gave me the phone number to the pulmonary doctor's office.

"In the meantime," he said, "just try and relax."

I told him I would and walked out. I made it to the car before I let go. I just could not help myself. I cried so hard and for so long. I just sat there thinking about my wife and kids. What were they going to do without me? I thought I could not drive. I felt like this was the end of my life. I was shaking; I was upset; and I was sad.

After about half an hour, my feelings changed. I dried my tears, and I was overwhelmed with anger and felt so much determination to fight and beat this. I was not going to let this be my ending. I called my wife at work. I asked for her and waited for her to pick up the line.

I said, "Hi, honey, you're not going to believe this. I have a tumor the size of a grapefruit in my right lung." That's what was causing the pain in my back.

I did the one thing I promised her I would never do. I broke her heart. I had tears running down my face a little and said, "Leslie, everything is going to be okay. I know the odds are not great. Somehow, I will survive this." I didn't know how to explain to her how I would survive this, but I just knew in my heart that I would.

Leslie said we would get through this. She went silent.

I said to her, "I am a fighter, and everything will be okay."

Leslie stayed pretty strong on the phone. I admired her strength!

I asked her to do me a favor. I said, "I need you to be strong for my girls and me. They will need you more than ever now. This is how we're going to look at this. Let's not cry until we have something to cry about. I'm still alive, and I will be strong for you in return. Please promise me this."

She agreed.

We hung up. Afterward Leslie told me she cried for a long time. I sat in my seat thinking about Leslie and our wedding day. It was a great day. I felt like the luckiest man in the world. I remembered our special vows to one another and my promise I made to her. I will only share this one part: "I will never break your heart." All of a sudden my comedian brothers came into my thoughts. Before my wedding they had put this bright white "HELP ME" on the bottom of my wing tip shoes. "HELP" on one and "ME" on the other. When I knelt down at the alter people began to laugh and the cameras went crazy.

All I could hear were clicking sounds and flash after flash! I thought, "Oh God." I remember looking over at Leslie saying, "Don't." She looked so frustrated. I shook my head back and forth at her and said in a whisper, "Uh huh, nope. It's not worth it." She smiled and stayed focused. Father Harding was a great sport about it as we discovered together what was so funny. He continued on without missing a beat. Afterward we all laughed together. I thought Leslie was all right, but she was so hurt from it. I just want to say I have patience, brothers! This thought made me smile, and I started the car and went to work. On the way in, I was thinking about our sick-leave option we have at the schools. I had never gone on a sick leave before, and I was nervous about it. I am not one to sit around much.

I told my coworkers what was going on and asked our day custodian about the sick bank. He was on the sick bank committee and knew the procedure to go out on sick leave, so it was explained to me. They all were shocked as well. I felt blessed to have a good job and health insurance.

I wanted to tell my girls the situation. I was so nervous. I did not want them to hurt anymore. After the divorce, the girls had gone through enough. I called them and asked to meet them for a family meeting.

The next morning we went to the hospital for the CAT scan. After it was over, we met back with Dr. Schwartz and talked about the results. Later that day Leslie and I drove out to meet the girls. When we got there, I called the girls to come out to the car to talk. They came out and climbed into the back of my car. They looked so scared. I just came out with it.

I said, "Girls, I have a large tumor in my right lung. I set up an appointment to meet the pulmonary specialist. He got us in right away. They will determine what kind of cancer I have and determine the best way to handle this. The doctor told me if they can remove it, then they will. We will have to see what happens from there. I want you to stay strong for Dad and look out for each other. I will keep you posted."

The girls wanted to go with us. I asked them if they had any questions. They both said no. As I looked at their eyes, they both had tears.

I said, "Let's not cry until we have something to cry about." In a soft voice, I said, "Dad's not dead, girls, just sick! Okay?"

They said okay.

I gave them a big hug and told them I loved them more than anything on this planet. We talked with them a little more, and then they went back inside the house. I felt so bad for them as we drove away. On the way home, it was pretty quiet in the car. Leslie asked me if I was okay. I said I was and that I was thinking about the time we met.

Life was great. I was thirty-eight years old. I had just gotten divorced. My baby girls were handling the divorce well. I was very proud of them. Divorce is not easy for most kids. I gave them a lot of reassurances that life would be okay. I told them Dad would always answer the phone, no matter what time of the day. And trust me, those babies put me to the test! About six months had passed, and I had gotten adjusted to my new single life. It was a great feeling to be free of that person's agony. I was thinking at the time what it would be like to really be in love, to meet someone whom you could share your thoughts with and all of your hopes and dreams.

I was telling my friends and family that love must only happen in Hollywood. I never thought it would happen to me. Just when you're not looking is when fate happens. My sister called and said it was time to move on.

She said, "You got your priorities straight, right?"

I said, "Right!"

"I think its time for you to date and move on with your life. I have a friend I would like you to meet."

I told her that I didn't think I was ready to meet anyone and that I had to be sure my head was on straight, and it wouldn't be fair to someone if it wasn't.

She laughed at me and said, "Does anyone have his or her head on straight?"

I said, "I don't know."

She said, "How would you ever know if you don't try?"

So I agreed to meet her friend. She gave me her phone number. Within a few days, I had called her.

I was really nervous until I heard her voice. It was like an angel was helping me be confident and strong. Within a few seconds, I was so relaxed, like it was destiny. She was very easy to talk to. We talked on the phone for hours. After two more days of talking on the phone with her, I couldn't believe my luck. I had called my sister back on Wednesday and was telling her how things were going and that I really enjoyed talking with her on the phone. I told her that we had planned to meet on Thursday evening for dinner if she and her husband could make it. It would make the evening less stressful, I thought, for both of us. She agreed. Everyone in the family was excited for us to get together; they all loved Leslie very much.

Thursday came fast. I left to go meet her at her place. I got there and knocked on the door. There was no sight of my sister and her husband anywhere, as usual. The girl would be late for her own funeral. "Sorry, Sis. You know I'm right!" When the door opened, I thought, Oh my God, I'm in deep. She was totally out-of-my-league beautiful. She had straight, blonde hair. Her eyes were so blue—like nothing I had ever seen. In that moment, I was thinking I had just met the woman of my dreams. She in every way was perfect for me. As I stared into those beautiful eyes, she introduced herself.

"Hi!" she said. "I'm Leslie."

She had a very beautiful smile. She had movie-star-perfect teeth. I paused for a second and said, "I'm Jim. It's very nice to meet you."

At that very moment, I did not care if my sister showed up at all. I knew the night would be fine. So she invited me in, and we sat down and talked for a while. She was extremely beautiful, that natural beautiful. She was very smart and well educated. She had a wonderful attitude toward life. It was that love that everyone searched for. I couldn't believe that this was happening to me. My heart felt more warmth and comfort than ever before. At that very moment, I knew that she was my soul mate and my search for love was over.

Within an hour, my sister showed up apologizing, and we ordered dinner from the local Chinese food restaurant. I was kind of new to the Asian food industry. So I asked Leslie for advice on what to order. I ended up ordering the orange chicken. Leslie ordered the cashew chicken, extra spicy. I really enjoyed the dinner and most of all being with my new soul mate. It was getting late, and I had to go to work the next morning at five a.m. My sister stayed to talk with Leslie. Leslie walked me to the door. We stepped outside the door and said our good-byes. It was the most special moment that two people in love could share: that first kiss!

I knew right there and then that I would marry this woman and spend the rest of my life with her. On my way home, I was sorting through my feelings. I had never felt this way about someone else before. I was so happy for a change. My heart felt safe and on the right path, nothing I ever felt in the past! My eyes started to water! I was crying. I was so happy! I thought then and there that no matter what happened, I had the courage to follow my heart and live my life for me for a change.

I wondered how my kids would do meeting her. How would they feel? Would they be mad at me? Hurt? Confused? We were soon going to find out! They met Leslie, and things worked out to be excellent for them. I was very happy for the girls. Anyway, we got home and watched some movies. Leslie and I spent the evening holding each other.

I had an appointment with the pulmonary doctor to meet him. Leslie's dad, stepmom, and my girls wanted to go and hear what he had to say. We all got there and were anxious to hear what was next. The doc came in the exam room and introduced himself.

"Hi! I am Dr. Belen." He began to explain the procedure. "James, as you know, you have a large, cancerous tumor in your right lung. What I will do is go down your throat and take some samples of the tumor. I want to do this right away."

Dr. Belen set up the bronchoscopy. After the bronchoscopy was over and the dust settled, we went back to Dr. Belen's office to get the results. Dr Belen explained that the tumor was large and was wrapped around my pulmonary artery.

"This will make it very difficult to remove. The type of cancer you have is non-small cell carcinoma. I felt at first this was a stage-three cancer with surgical options, but now I feel this is a stage-four cancer because of the location and size. There is no room to clamp off the pulmonary artery."

The room went silent. My first thought was, I am no medical expert, but I do know what stage-four cancer is.

In case you don't know, it's the worst cancer to get. It's usually inoperable and with not-good results. Death usually occurs, was my next thought. My heart just fell to the floor. I tried not to show any emotion and to stay strong. I looked at my wife and Mom and Dad. I smiled at them. My eyes were overwhelmed with tears.

I asked, "What are the chances to survive this?"

Dr. Belen said in a soft voice, "I don't know." He thought for a moment. "Maybe you have a ten to fifteen percent chance to survive this. The odds are against you. I'm sorry, James, but you will need to talk with a surgeon to see if it's even possible to operate on."

After a moment of processing the news, I said, "Okay, then that's what I will do." I smiled at him and said, "Thank you."

I stayed positive! I said to my family, "It's going to be okay. I got the number to the surgeon, and we will call to set up an appointment. Come on, let's go eat."

Later I went to work and picked up the sick-bank papers to be filled out by my doctor. I took the copy of the CAT scan to work to show my coworkers. I spoke with the day custodian about our sick-leave policy and asked how much sick time was left in our sick bank. He was not sure. My coworkers were very surprised by the size of the tumor. They all wished me good luck and asked me to stay in touch and to keep them posted. During the week, I had Dr. Schwartz fill out the sick-bank papers and handed them back into my work. At the time, I was grateful to have benefits from work.

About a week had passed, and we got in to see the surgeon. He came in the room and introduced himself.

"Hi, I am Dr. Apostolou."

He was a very confident doctor and well respected for his work. He was very straightforward with the outlook of the situation. "James," he said, "this doesn't look good for you. You see, after examining your CAT scan and reviewing your bronchoscopy, this tumor is very large. It's wrapped around your pulmonary artery and has grown through the back of your lung and through the front as well. I don't feel it's operable at this time. If I made an attempt to operate now, the odds would be against you."

My wife asked, "What kind of odds are we talking?"

He said, "About ten to fifteen percent. You see, there is not enough room to clamp off your pulmonary artery. It's very possible that you will bleed out on the table. You would need to do the radiation treatment and chemo first. I mean sixty days straight of radiation and three months of a very aggressive chemo treatment. Then we will see if it shrinks enough to operate on. Your chances for survival will be better if it shrinks. You will have at least a twenty percent chance then."

I was so blown away by what I was hearing. My wife had tears in her eyes. My in-laws were just stunned. I looked at my wife and said, "So we do the treatment. Everything will be okay!" I looked at Dr. Apostolou. "Twenty percent is pretty good, right?"

I just smiled at him and then to my wife. She was so hurt. When I looked back at her, she looked just crushed. I said thank you to Dr. Apostolou and said we would be in touch.

We shook hands. We gathered our things and left. Leslie had to go to work, and my in-laws drove me home. As Leslie left, I watched her leave. She started to cry some more. I felt so helpless. I wish I could help her, I thought.

As I stood on the sidewalk watching her drive away, Leslie's dad said in a soft voice, "Come on, son, let's go home."

I wiped the tears from my eyes, turned around, and went with them. As we walked to the car I looked up at dad and thought about his situation with colon cancer and how he was dealing with it. He had already developed side effects like neuropathy and memory loss.

I did not say much on the way home. All I could think about was how hurt my wife was. When we got back to my place, I thanked Mom and Dad for driving me home and went in the house. I had to call and schedule appointments with the oncology doctor and the radiation-oncologist doctor. At this point, I was thinking, How much worse can things get? When I called the oncology doctor, he wanted to see me first before going to the radiation doctor.

Leslie came home, and I just hugged her for a long time. We ate dinner and talked for a while. It felt strange to talk about death and putting things in order in case I died. I wanted to remind her who to call to receive my benefits and insurance. I gave her those numbers to call in the event of my death. I asked her to look out for my little girls, especially my youngest. She just loved Leslie and looked up to her. Leslie was frustrated talking about this. After all, it did feel like a bad dream. However, it was something I had to talk about.

Shortly after our arrival at the doctor's office, we were called back to the exam room. The doctor and staff there were very nice.

The doctor introduced himself. "Hi. I'm Dr. Schwartz. How are you?"

The answer is yes, I have two doctors with the same last name. He was very confident and sure of himself. I admired this; it was the combination I was looking for. To me if he did not possess these two, we were all done. Nobody wants a weak doctor, right? I felt so comfortable with him and the staff that I decided to stay with him for treatment.

The doc started to explain what was happening to me and was amazed at my current condition. He asked me how long my knees and ankles were swelled up. I told him since the spring of 2009. He asked me about my fingers and how long had they been this way. I told him the same, since this spring.

He said to me, "Why didn't you go to your doctor?"

I smiled and told him a short story about what I had been through. After the story, he looked at me and said he was sorry to hear this. He knew of this doctor.

I smiled at him and told him, "At this point, I wouldn't change anything, and I am in good hands now. Let's focus on moving forward.

He said, "Very well, that's what we will do." He stated that he spoke with the surgeon and came up with a plan of attack that should work for me.

He started to tell us what chemo was and the side effects that most people got. I was thinking to myself of all the bad luck that I have, and I would probably be that guy who gets all the side effect problems. However, another day with my family was a fair trade, regardless what happened. I loved my wife and children and my family. I loved my life and what it had to offer. There is no greater feeling than love; if you don't have it, you better find it before your time expires!

The plan was to give me the strongest chemo they had for three days in a row, then twenty-one days of rest.

I asked the doctor about side effects. The doctor explained that with every person, the side effects were different. He said everyone reacted differently to the chemo. We would have to see what happened and see what I could handle. He said, "Any other questions?"

The room was quiet.

He said, "It was very nice to meet you and your family. Take care, James, and we will see you on Monday."

I thanked the doctor and staff, and we left. On the way over to the hospital, I stated that I liked that doctor and staff, and I wanted to stay there for treatment. I explained to my family about how important it was to me to have a doctor who's confident. My wife and in-laws thought he was a confident doctor as well. My appointment with the radiation doctor was scheduled the same day as the oncology doctor. We headed over to the DMC Huron Valley Karmanos cancer center to meet the doctor and staff. We walked in and were greeted by the receptionist.

As we waited in the lobby, I was observing how things ran there. They had a special parking lot for the cancer patients that was right next to the building. They had a large coin dispenser at the reception desk for patients to take to get out of the security gate. As we continued to wait, about three people forgot coins as they left and had to walk back in order to get them so they could leave.

Dad said, "You might want to grab a handful, son."

I just smiled and gave him the nod. I asked dad how he was doing.

He said, "One day at a time."

I said, "I admire your courage and strength, Dad. I bet you never thought you would have a cancer buddy when you got diagnosed, did you?"

Dad smiled.

I yelled out, "I love you, Daddy." Other patients just stared at us. Dad was shaking his head back and forth feeling embarrassed. I love picking on him a little. It keeps him sharp.

Like I said earlier, Dad had colon cancer and was going through hell already. When Leslie called him to tell him that his best son had a cancer tumor, he just went silent about a moment. He continued to listen to her explain and did not say much except he wanted to go with us to all the doctor appointments. I felt that Dad is a real man with old-fashioned values. Respect, honor, and trust are how he lives his life. I was built the same way. I think this is why we get along so well.

We definitely have a great father and son-in-law relationship. It was important for me to stay strong and keep a positive attitude for Dad. After a few minutes, they called us back to the exam room. A couple of minutes had passed, and the radiation doctor came in with a social worker to talk with us. She introduced herself.

"Hi, I am Dr. Hart, and this is our social worker." She shook our hands, and then she began to explain about radiation and what to expect from it. "James, I have talked with the surgeon and oncology doctor, and they feel the same as I do about taking an aggressive approach. You have a very large tumor in there. It's attached to your chest cavity in two locations, and if it does start to shrink, it will be painful for you as it tears away from your chest cavity. We plan to get it as small as we can so we can surgically remove it. About halfway through the sixty days, we will do another CAT scan to see its progress. We will be setting up an alignment tattoo that is very small and hardly noticeable. This will enable our technicians to align the area in question and give the appropriate amount of radiation. Today, I would like you to meet our social worker and talk with her."

She introduced the social worker doctor and said, "I will see you on Monday," and left the room.

The social worker wanted to know how I was handling the situation. I told her that I was doing okay. I said, "I am a very strong person, both physically and mentally. I will fight this until I cannot fight anymore. I do realize what has happened to me, and I do realize what treatment is in store for me. I am scared a little. Some things are out of our control. I am more scared for my wife and my daughters."

The doctor said she could understand that. The doctor asked to speak with Leslie in private.

While I was waiting there, I tried to put myself in Leslie's shoes for a moment to try and see and understand what she was going through. I wish I could help her, I thought. My only ideas were to stay focused and positive for her. I was thinking about my wife's other side of the family. She was also from a divorced family, and her mom and two sisters were, let's say, difficult to get along with. It's the Cinderella story; that's for sure. I have never seen so much jealousy out of three people in my lifetime.

Anyway, this was one of my worries. Here, I had been blessed with the greatest woman in the world and then got this cancer just five years later. I just slid back in the chair, looking up at the ceiling and talking to God. I yelled to God, "I love life! Who loves life more than me?"

I said to God in a low whisper, "God, what did I do wrong?" My eyes began to water. I said, "I walk your path. I am a man of honor, truth, respect, and trust! I have given and shown these words to my children. I mean, what the hell did I do? Tell me so I can fix it," I said a little louder. I got out some tissues and cleaned myself up. I never got an answer! About ten minutes later, Leslie came out and seemed to be okay.

I was relieved to see her smile a little. I waited until we got in the car to ask if she was all right. As soon as my backside hit the seat, I said, "Are you okay?"

She said she was extremely worried about me and wanted to talk some more with the doctor.

I said, "That's all right. That is what they are there for."

I didn't have the courage to ask what they talked about. I thought to myself, I will show her how strong I really am and stay positive through this. After a couple of minutes, I said, "I love you more than anything on this planet."

She smiled and said she loved me too.

We lived five minutes from the hospital. I just held her hand and was quiet the rest of the way home.

We got back to the house to let the puppies out. I have two male black Labradors and a bichon poodle mix. The bichon's name is Ally; she looks like a Sesame Street character, and the labs are Chewie and Sage. Chewie has been the most troublesome dog. He has been through three cages and the garage door, and the list goes on. Sage, on the other hand, has been an angel sent from the heavens. Ally is just the most adorable puppy you will ever see.

Anyway, those are my puppies. The pups were outside running around in the backyard. I walked over to my wife and gave her a big hug and started to sing to her, "Don't worry about a thing, because every little thing's going to be all right!" It is a Bob Marley song. We just slowly danced as I sang the rest of it.

We spent the rest of the weekend talking about Monday. I was nervous about taking chemo and starting the sixty days of radiation. The fear of the unknown is so powerful. On Sunday, I was reminding Leslie that if I died, I had some insurance through my work to pay for the funeral, and I reminded her about the contact numbers. This was a hard thing to talk about. Leslie was a little mad at me, but I had to face the reality of the situation. I said, "Leslie! I love you, and it's just in case."

She just nodded to me.

I smiled at her and continued to smile until I got a smile back, even if it had tears in it. We had some General Hospital to catch up on, so we went to the family room to watch our favorite recorded soap.

Monday morning came quickly, and we were on our way to the oncology doctors for chemo. The first day was eight hours of chemo. Prior to this visit, they gave me a medication prescription to help with the nausea. I was thinking to myself, This just doesn't look good.

We got there, and they called us to come back right away. We were walking back to the exam room when I felt overwhelmed with anxiety, like I was signing my own death warrant.

I did not say a word to my wife because she was so stressed out. I just said to myself, Suck it up, big boy, and get in the chair.

The nurse introduced herself. "Hi! I am Karen, and I will be handling your chemo treatments, okay?"

She was so nice and patient. I listened to her instructions for overnight care of the PICC line. They were leaving the PICC line in overnight because I had to come back the next two days. She started to tell me about the chemos they were going to give me. This chemo is one of the strongest chemos they make.

"It does give people side effects," she said.

I told her that we talked about it with Dr. Schwartz, and he explained everything. After a couple of minutes, I said it took all the strength I had to come here today.

I felt like I was signing my life away. Karen said she could understand that. "Chemo is a big deal, James, but when it's your only option to live, you do what must be done!"

"Right," I said. "Right!"

I reached over and turned the TV on for some noise. It was so quiet in there. I could not take my eyes off my wife; she looked so afraid and cheated. I just smiled at her and said, "Everything is going to be all right." Leslie and I talked about life and family.

Leslie said, "I don't know what Chewie would do without you."

I just smiled. I said, "That little guy has put us through some hell."

We just laughed about all the crazy things that dog had done to us. That's a whole new book in itself. Move over, Marley. Chewie's coming!

Karen had introduced us to some other patients that were their getting chemo. One lady had the same thing I did but not as aggressive. Another gentleman had colon cancer like Dad. There were others there as well with breast cancer. I looked at them for a while; they all lost their hair. Some seemed as if they had given up on life and were depressed. They were just lying there, hoping to die. I thought to myself, I am not going to end up this way! Hell no!

I could deal with the bald head and hairless body, but I refused to be defeated! One of the women I spoke with still worked at her office job. She asked what I did for a living. I told her. She said she could not see me going back to my line of work with that strong of a chemo. She said I would know by tonight how I would do! Right then I decided I needed a private room from that day forward. If I was going to beat cancer, it was not going to be in a negative environment! Positive! Positive! Positive!

There was nothing wrong with the community room; I could have survived it out there, but I am a private-room kind of guy. It was hard to be around people who were negative all the time. After six hours, it was all I could do with the negative attitudes. I told these people that to me, life was awesome! What I was listening to was just ridiculous to me. You have your freedom to do what you want. You have all of these great pleasures to enjoy that God gave you. I mean, I got out, and I enjoyed life to its fullest.

I was not giving up. I said to the women, "What about love? Have you not experienced that?"

She said, "Once," and then she smiled.

I must have jogged an old memory she had. If I could give back to the cancer population and have my chance to speak to them, it would be these words in this whole book. Stay positive at all times. Focus on healing. Live your life and enjoy each day God gives you, even if it's only one more day.

After the eight hours were over, we were off to the hospital for radiation. I was feeling a little nauseated when we left. However, the pills they gave seemed to be helping me a little. We got there and did not have to wait very long. When we were called back, we were introduced to a few more members of the radiation team. Everyone was easygoing and welcoming. I liked the staff there right away. The technician asked how chemo went.

I told her, "So far, I am okay."

She said I would know by tonight how I would handle it and to just hang in there.

I just smiled and said okay. I thought to myself, That's the third or fourth time I have heard that today.

The radiation was a painless treatment. They radiated through the front and the back of my chest. I just lay there, and the machine did all the work. After a few minutes, I was done.

She said, "See how easy it is?"

I said, "Yes, I do. I will see you tomorrow."

Leslie and I were on our way to the parking lot. We jumped in the car and were headed home. As we approached the security gate, my wife said, "It requires coins."

I said, "I got this," and pulled out the handful of coins Dad told me to get at our first appointment.

See, kids, if you listen to your father, life will be much easier.

Anyway, we were on our way home. Day one was done. I was really tired and went to lie down on the coach. I was doing okay. I was a little nervous about what was in store for me later but thought it was out of my control now. I asked Leslie if we could just order a pizza for dinner, and she agreed. I ordered from our favorite local place. They said forty-five minutes. So I took a catnap until it came.

I love pizza. It's all four food groups in one in my eyes. When the doorbell rang, I woke up right away and paid the delivery guy. I was glad I had an appetite after our crazy day at the doctor's. We ate dinner and talked for a while. I asked Leslie if I looked okay to her. Leslie said I did. However, on the inside, I was wishing I had not eaten so much food. I said I was going to lie back down. I felt so tired and weak. I went in the bedroom and put on some sweats and climbed back on the couch to sleep some more.

Leslie said, "While you sleep, I am going down to the family room to watch my soaps."

I said, "Okay. Don't watch General Hospital though."

She said she had other soaps she recorded to watch.

I fell asleep. After a couple of hours of rest, I sat up and turned the TV on. I felt so sick. My ear was ringing a little, and I felt so nauseated and dizzy. I went to the bathroom to take a hot shower in hopes that it would make me feel a little better. After the shower, I just climbed in to bed to rest some more. About an hour had passed, and Leslie came upstairs to see how I was doing. I was telling her how cold I was and that I was a little lightheaded. I said my ear started ringing and would not stop. Ringing in your ear is so annoying. Leslie got me some more blankets and covered me up. I lay there awhile and fell asleep.

I woke up in the middle of the night so sick. I got up and ran into the bathroom. After a run of diarrhea and throwing up, I jumped back in the shower to get warmed up. As I stood in the shower, I thought to myself, What an idiot I was to eat so much. I felt so cold that even the hot water could not warm me up. Leslie came in there and was asking me if I was okay.

With my teeth chattering like crazy, I said, "I am. I'm just cold."

Leslie said, "I will get you a towel." She brought it back in the bathroom and said, "I will get you the heating pad for the bed. It will help you get warm."

I said, "Okay, babe," and smiled at her. I climbed out of the shower and got dressed. I went in the kitchen to get my nausea medication out of my coat pocket.

I took the pills and went back to lie down. Leslie made up the bed with the heat pad. The pad warmed me up fast. I was feeling so dehydrated and weak. I drank some water and finally went back to sleep. The morning came, and it was time to get up for my second round of chemo. Leslie's dad and mom were coming to pick me up to take me. I got up and got back in the shower before Leslie left for work. I was feeling pretty sick to my stomach still and did not want to eat. I said good-bye to my beautiful bride as she headed off for the day.

Right after I got dressed, Mom and Dad came in to get me. They asked how I was doing. I said I was feeling sick. I decided to take the next nausea pill just before we left. I was so grateful to have Dad and Mom in my life. Dad was a strong person and cast a large shadow. Mom was the same. I thought to myself that I hoped I had time left to show them that I was a great son. I told them on the way there that I loved their daughter more than anything.

I said, "I just want you guys to know how appreciated you are as well. I am very grateful for everything you have done for me."

As sick as I felt, I was not sure what was going to happen to me after the second dose of chemo. We got there, and I said good morning to Penny. We sat down and waited to be called back. I was telling Mom and Dad that they had only one private room back there, and I was going to ask for it from this day forward. I said that I would like my privacy while going through this. The rest of the chairs back there were lined up side by side in a community room.

We were called back, and I said good morning to Melanie and Karen. They asked how my first night went. I told them, "It was a little rough, but before I tell you about it, can I ask you a favor?"

Karen said sure.

I said, "I was hoping to get the private room from this day forward, if that would not be too much trouble."

Karen said, "Of course you could have it."

I said thank you to her, and we headed in there. I finished telling her about my night.

She smiled and said, "You hang in there."

I said okay.

She brought in an extra chair for Dad to sit in. I was telling them that I was afraid to eat again after my night.

Karen happened to overhear us talking and said, "No matter what happens, you have to force yourself to eat, and drink a lot of fluids. Do you understand? You will be a lot worse off if you get dehydrated. They will admit you in the hospital. Drink as much as you can."

It was the way she said it that had my full attention. The word "hospital" was echoing in my head over and over. That was all I had to hear. I was not staying in the hospital. I asked for water or juice, please! Karen came back to hook me up to the IV and brought some water back with her.

Dad, Mom, and I all talked for a while. I finished telling them about yesterday's experience. I told them about the other patients that were there that seemed depressed and did not seem to care if they lived or died. I said to them, "Staying focused on the positive and enjoying what's left of your life is really what's important. Being this sick, everything is not about money now, is it?

They said, "No, it's not."

We talked about the family and life and the impact the illness had made. I was listening to Dad talk about his cancer and his surgery. He was telling us about his chemo port they installed and how tender his chest felt. He said he couldn't wait for his chemo treatments to be over. He was tired of being sick.

I said, "Dad, you're doing well. You have inspired me to fight and appreciate life more. Not that I didn't already." I just smiled at him. I was worried about him. I said, "Do you remember the time Leslie had her surgery?"

Mom said, "Which time?"

I said, "The one where the pretty nurse complimented Dad's pink bag."

Dad smiled.

The story goes like this: Leslie had her surgery. We—Mom, Dad, and I—were on our way to visit Leslie, and Dad and Mom were helping me carry Leslie's luggage. I gave Dad the pink bag to carry. We made it up to Leslie's floor and had a long walk to go. A pretty nurse caught up to us as we were walking, and I asked her if she wouldn't mind participating in a joke.

I said, "All I need is for you to catch up to the gentleman there and compliment his pink bag. He is my dad!"

She laughed at first and then said, "Okay, I will do it!"

She caught up to Dad and said, "Sir, that's a beautiful pink bag you have there!"

Dad just shook his head. I could hear him say, "That guy back there put you up to this, didn't he?"

The morning seemed to go by fast. Karen came back and unplugged my IV and said, "You're all done."

I said thank you to her, and I said I would see her tomorrow.

She gave me a hug and said, "Hang in there."

The second day of chemo was done, and we were on our way to radiation. We got there and went back to the small waiting area for the radiation patients. It was set up real nice. They had a nice-sized table there with a thousand-piece puzzle to work on while we waited. On the walls in the little waiting area were glued together puzzles put into frames. They were the puzzles the other cancer patients put together over the past few years.

They called me back for my treatment. I removed my shirt and climbed onto the table. They adjusted my alignment, and the technician left the room and shut the large door.

The machine turned on, and after a few seconds, it rotated to my backside. After about one minute, the treatment was over. I was thinking while I lay on the table looking around how amazing science was and what science can do these days. The treatment was over, and we headed out. I said thank you to everyone and left for home.

I was back at home, lying on the couch. Dad had stayed with me to keep an eye on me. We started to watch a western, The Good, the Bad, and the Ugly. It was one of our favorites.

I had fallen asleep, and when I woke up about an hour later, Dad had fallen asleep too. I restarted the movie and went to the restroom. On the way back, I stopped by the kitchen to get something to drink. Dad had woken up and said he missed the movie. I said I did too, and I had reset it to the beginning. I came back and grabbed one of Grandma's old quilts and got comfy on the couch. I drank some juice and ate some leftover pizza from the day before. The movie had restarted, and about twenty minutes into it, I fell asleep again. Dad did too; I woke up an hour later to go to the bathroom again, and he was asleep too. I laughed to myself. That chemo makes you urinate a lot.

I came back in the living room and restarted the movie for the third time. Dad woke up for the third time and asked if he missed it. I said no and that it was just starting.

He looked at me for a moment and said in a firm voice, "I'm watching you, son."

I started to laugh and said I had fallen asleep again too. We both started to laugh. We both stayed awake this time to watch the whole thing. Hey, I don't mean any disrespect, Clint. You're still my hero.

After the movie was over, Dad headed home. Just before he walked out, he said he was going to take me the next day to chemo. I said I would see him in the morning then. I thought about Karen, the nurse, telling me to eat and drink. I had to force myself to eat. Everything tasted like metal though. I got up to make a fried egg sandwich. It seemed to be the only thing that sounded okay to eat. I grabbed a bottle of juice to drink.

Leslie came home, and we talked and hugged for a while. She felt bad that she had to work and could not be there to take me to the chemo doctor. I told her not to worry, that I was doing okay, and that Dad and I had fun watching movies. I started to laugh because of what happened. I told Leslie the story, and by the time I got to the third-attempt-to-watch-it part, she was laughing.

I was really tired and went back to the couch to lie down. I had forgotten to take the nausea medication and started to feel real sick. I took the medication and lay down for a while. After a couple of hours of sleep, it started all over again; I was cold and had massive diarrhea. I went back into the shower to get warm. This time I just slid down into the tub and ran the hot water for a while.

As I was sitting in the tub under the hot water, it helped me to think about great moments I had in my life. I started to think about when my kids were born and the excitement I felt as a new father. When my oldest daughter was born, she changed my life forever. I went from a wild gypsy soul straight into totally responsible parent mode and have not quit yet. I remember walking into the nursery and giving the nurse my ID. The nurse took me over to her room of rocking chairs.

"Please sit here, and I will bring her to you."

I said okay, and the nurse came back with my little girl.

When I held her for the first time, I said something to her that no one knows about, until now. My own daughter will learn of this for the first time when she reads this book. I said in a soft voice, "Dad will love you forever. I promise to you that I will always be here for you and look after you until God calls for me. You don't now how lucky you are to have me for a dad. We will have as much fun as we can while you grow up. Enjoy life to the fullest!"

I just hugged her for a while until the nurse came back to check on her. The nurse picked her up and took her back to her temporary bed for her to sleep. I felt so proud and honored for the chance to be a father. Even to this day, I have always been there for them both.

I got out of the shower and dried off. I put on some sweats and some warm socks. I looked at my beautiful wife and said I was okay. She just smiled. She asked me if I wanted the heating pad again.

I said, "Yes, please."

I just climbed in to bed. It was another rough night. The ringing in my ear seemed to get louder, and my hearing began to change for the worse in the same ear. I was so glad the nausea medication started to work though. I remember asking God for a break on the diarrhea, please. "My bottom is burning!" I said. He must have been listening, because I made it through the night.

The next morning came fast, and I got up before Leslie had to leave for work so I could take a shower. As I was getting dressed, she was telling me how proud she was of me to fight this.

I said thank you to her and gave her a big hug and kiss. I said, "Thank you for everything." I was so grateful to have her in my life. I said, "Have a good day, and I will talk to you soon."

Dad came to pick me up, and we were on are way to the doc's office for the third round of chemo.

He asked me how the night went; I said about the same. I said I stayed on top of the nausea meds this time. The diarrhea was not so bad this time either. We got in to the doc's office and said good morning to Penny. Melanie called me back right away. Melanie had to draw some more blood samples to test. I had to pass my white-blood count before she could give me the last dose of chemo. After the blood was drawn and the results came back, I was all set for my third round. We headed back to the room.

Dad and I talked about the place where Dad goes fishing every year. He was saying how beautiful it was there and how I would love it there too. I listened to Dad talk about the great fishing spot for a while. Dad was good at distracting me. I'm sure I looked a little stressed. It helped me a lot to get the chemo off my mind anyway. Leslie made Dad and me a day-bag loaded with goodies. This also helped take my mind off chemo. We shared some treats with Karen and other patients. The chemo treatment seemed to pass quickly with the help of Dad and Leslie's treat bag. Karen came in the room and removed the stent from my chest.

"All right," she said, "you are all set to go. You have an appointment with the doc next week to see how you're doing."

I told her I would be there.
She asked me if I was okay.
I said, "I am okay. I am just tired."
She gave me a hug and said, "See you in a week."
I said good-bye to everyone and left.

Dad and I were on our way to the hospital for the radiation treatment. When we got there, Dr. Hart said she wanted to talk with me afterward. So I got through the radiation treatment, and they put me in an exam room. Dr. Hart came in and took a quick look at me to see how I was doing. She said that I looked good and seemed to be doing okay. They gave me a card for the valet parking.

I said, "I do not need that. Please give it to someone else that's worse off, please."

She said, "Just in case, for those real cold days."

I said thank you and accepted the card because I was so damn cold all the time. We were on the way out, and Dad said it was a very nice gift. He said that they didn't treat him that well at the hospital where he got treatment. I told him I was sorry to hear that. I just smiled. We got into the car to leave.

We got up to the gate, and Dad looked over at me and said, "You remembered the coins, right?"

"Of course I did," I said.

I handed Dad a few extra coins to keep for next time. Dad said to me, "At least two of my kids listen when I speak."

I just smiled at Dad.

We were on our way to get some breakfast. We decided to go to Woody's in Walled Lake. It's a great place to eat for breakfast or lunch. After our great breakfast, we went back to my house to rest for a while. I threw in the next movie: Two Mules for Sister Sara. It was another great western with Clint Eastwood. I thought to myself, Life is still good. I'm here another day.

After the movie was over, Dad headed home, and it was time for me to get some more sleep. Leslie came home soon, and we were eating dinner. I decided not to eat so much this time after going by what I went through the other two nights. My attitude was: Whatever happens, I will get through it! I felt very weak and decided to grab Grandma's old quilt and lie on the couch for a while.

As the night approached, I felt worse and soon found myself back in the shower again. My teeth were chattering so loud and hard that I wondered if other people ever broke a tooth. I turned the handle over to hot. I sat there thinking about my kids. I was wondering how they were doing. I remembered this time when my oldest daughter was four years old. She wanted a baby sister so badly. She came up to me in the living room one day and was staring at me with a very cute smile.

I looked back at her and said, "Hi!"

She said hi back, still smiling at me.

"What are you doing in your room?" I asked.

"Just thinking, Dad."

"What are you thinking about?"

She came right out with it and said, "Dad, I would like to have a baby sister."

"Really?"

"I need someone to play with and talk to."

"Having a baby sister is a big responsibility," I said. "They're messy and they throw up, and you have to change diapers."

She said, "I know, but I still want one." She started begging me to get her one, like I could just drive to the local toy store and pick one up off the shelf. "Please, Daddy! Please, Daddy!"

I said I would have to talk with Mom first.

She said okay and walked back to her room.

I sat there just kind of laughing to myself. Then I realized where she got the idea. Her little friend just had a baby brother. She was probably saying how cool it was to feed him and help keep him clean. I got up and walked to my daughter's room and pushed the door the rest of the way open. She was sitting in her little chair looking at a book.

I asked, "Did you get this idea from your little friend?"

"We were talking about her brother," she said, "and you know how much I like my dolls."

"Yes, I do. All right, if you're willing to help take care of a new baby, I will talk with your mom."

My daughter said, "Dad, where do babies come from?"

I said, "Kmart layaway?" I said it so smoothly that I believed it at first. It was all I could come up with at the time.

That topic was never brought up again, thank God. At the time, I could only hope that she would forget my lie. I didn't know what else to say, so I left it at that. She got her wish about a year later. When we brought the youngest daughter home, my oldest was doing okay until the youngest threw up on her.

The hot water ran cold. I thought, Why can't someone invent a water heater that has an endless supply of hot water? That would be kick-ass for cancer patients.

I climbed back in to bed and got some sleep.

THE MIRACLE

The next morning I decided that every day I was going to take showers before Leslie left for work, no matter how I felt, even if I was going to sit in the chair in the living room. I don't know about you, but for me, taking showers seemed to give me a sense of normalcy. It was how I started my day. It also helped me preserve my dignity. It also gave me hope that my life would return back to normal someday.

Dad was coming to take me to my radiation appointment because I felt so run down. Over the next two weeks, I had developed a major hearing loss, and the ringing in my ears was so bad. I also had developed neuropathy problems in my feet and hands. My body was itching all over, and I was losing hair so fast. I had shaved my head bald. I lost all my hair, including my eyelashes. But you know what? I still was glad to be alive. I didn't look so bad bald either. Leslie went out and bought me a couple of hats to wear.

Over the next few weeks, I was taking things one day at a time. I still had radiation treatments to go to and follow-up appointments with all of my doctors. I spent a lot of time talking on the phone with family and friends. I felt very lucky to have the support I had.

I had to go see a hearing doctor to evaluate the hearing loss. After the hearing test, I had lost 40 percent of my hearing in my right ear. He could not help me with the ringing issue. He referred me to a hearing specialist in Waterford, Michigan. I set up an appointment to go see her.

Twenty-one days went by fast, and it was time for round two of chemo. I was talking with the oncology doctor, Dr. Schwartz. I was telling him about some of the side effects I had from the strong chemo. As we talked some more, he decided it would be best if he switched to a different kind of chemo. I was grateful that I had choices still. He asked me how everything else was doing. I said I'm staying positive, doc. I asked Dr. Schwartz about having a port installed. I had had enough of the needle pokes already, I said.

He said, "James, you will have to set that up with the surgeon."

"Okay, I will call him."

Dr. Schwartz asked me, "How is life?"

I told him that even though I had these issues and all these side effect problems, I was still glad to be alive. I smiled at him.

"You hang in there, James," he said, "and call me if there are any problems."

It was time for the eight-hour chemo treatment. I felt so tired and weak. Dad and Mom Dopke were with me. I was telling Mom and Dad about how I was feeling. I said, "Chemo is a lot tougher than I thought."

Dad said, "It sure is."

"Either way, I still have to keep fighting" I said'.

I was walking back to the reception area and saw Penny. She was on the phone when we came in. She asked how I was doing. I smiled at her and said the truth.

"I am very tired and weak, and I hope God is looking out for me."

Penny smiled and said, "It will be okay."

I smiled at her. I was waiting to see Melanie to do the blood work. Everything came back positive, and we went in the back to my private suite. I said good morning to Karen and asked how she was doing.

She said she was doing great. She asked the question, "How are you doing?"

"I'm tired," I said, "and I feel weak but ready to continue the fight."

"That's normal after taking that strong of chemo. You are here, James. You may be tired, but you look good. Your blood work looks great. Have a seat, and we will get started."

I sat in the recliner. I asked Karen, "Instead of the PICC line, could I have an IV?"

She said, "That's fine. You know I will have to poke you again tomorrow."

"I know," I said.

"Okay," she said, and she got started.

We were talking about Christmas. Dad and Mom Dopke were talking about canceling Christmas at their house on Christmas Eve. Mom felt with Dad and I being sick, it would be best. I smiled at Mom and said, "You guys do what works for you. As sick as I am, I don't plan on going anywhere anyway. Don't cancel Christmas because of me. What about all the other family members that look forward to Christmas with Grandma?"

Mom said, "This is true," and smiled at me.

I said, "I will miss everyone, but my presence is not too cheerful. I don't want to ruin anyone's holidays. I will be fine at home."

Most of the day, I kept my thoughts to myself. I listened to Mom and Dad talk about the holidays. I kept thinking about my girls and my family and hoped that they were doing okay. The eight hours of chemo were over, and Karen was removing the IV. Karen reached over and kissed my bald head. I stood up and gave her a hug.

I said, "Thank you for everything that you do. What would this world be like without great people like you?"

She smiled and said in a joking manner, "Get out of here."

I put on my coat and loaded up my goodies, and we were off to the hospital for radiation. We got downstairs to the main entrance, and you could hear the wind howling outside. Last year I went out and bought a large North Face parka. This thing is great and definitely keeps you warm. I zipped up my zipper all the way to my chin and flipped up my hood and said, "Okay, I am ready."

Dad and Mom laughed at me.

Dad said, "You look like that little kid from The Christmas Story. You know, the little boy that says, 'I can't put my arms down.' His mom had bundled him up in layers of clothes. The boy could barely move."

At least I made somebody laugh today, I thought. I said to Dad, "Where is the car?"

Dad smiled, and we all walked out together. We headed over to the hospital for my radiation treatment. We all said hello to the receptionist and walked back to the waiting room. The technician came to get me. The radiation treatment was over, and we were headed home. I thanked Mom and Dad for taking me.

Dad said he would take me tomorrow. I said okay. I got home and let the puppies run for a while. I walked in the living room and lay down on the couch to rest. I was not trying to fall asleep so I could let the puppies in. Just as I started to nod off, Chewie was scratching at the door. I got up to go let them in. I went back to the couch and Grabbed grandma's old, comfy quilt.

The puppies and I all curled up together and took a nap for a few hours. I woke to the sound of the dogs barking at their mommy coming home. Leslie came into the house, and we all greeted her at the door.

"Welcome home," I said, like I had not seen her in a month.

I was hugging her, and the puppies were jumping on her. She asked how chemo went. I said fine. I told Leslie about how Mom and Dad Dopke wanted to cancel their Christmas Eve party. I told Leslie that I planned on staying home regardless what happened. I was not feeling bad about myself.

I said that I just felt it would be best if I stayed home. Leslie did not agree. Her feelings were hurt. I said, "If they plan to still have the party, it would be okay if you and the girls wanted to go. I am totally okay with that."

Leslie said, "Not a chance! I am staying right here with you."

She smiled at me and reached over to give me a kiss. I kissed her back. I smiled at Leslie and just stared into her eyes. She asked me what I wanted for dinner.

I said, "How about pizza?"

She said, "That sounds good," and smiled at me. At this point I knew Leslie was tired of pizza, but she knew it was all I could handle. She had so much support for me. God bless her!

The pizza was delivered, and we sat down to eat. We talked some more about Christmas at Dad's. Leslie was really upset about it. I told her that everything would be fine if she and the girls still wanted to go. Leslie said no.

I said, "Okay, we will have fun here."

I went in the living room and sat in the recliner. I covered myself up with a quilt that Leslie's grandma made. For some reason I took a huge liking to this certain quilt. I called it "my healing blanket." When I told Leslie about my feelings toward the quilt she smiled and said, "It was my grandma's favorite. Grandma would have loved the fact that you like it because it was one that she made herself."

I said, "If you can hear me, Grandma, thank you for the quilt. I am very grateful."

Leslie went downstairs to do some chores while I slept. About an hour had passed, and I got up to go stretch out in bed.

I fell asleep for a few hours and woke up to my teeth chattering and a soaked bed. I was sweating so bad that the bed was soaked from head to toe. I got up and went into the shower to get warm. Leslie woke up and changed the bedding so I would not feel bad. She had it all done by the time I came back. I was sitting in the shower and letting the hot water come down on me. I was so cold. My teeth were chattering so loud. Right away, I started to think about something to take my mind off being sick.

I was thinking about my oldest daughter when she was five years old. It was summertime, and I was in the kitchen cleaning up after dinner when she came in there and tugged on my leg.

Totally serious, she said, "Dad, there's a boogeyman in my room, and he won't leave."

I said, "Really? That's not good!"

She said, "Make him go away."

I reached down to grab her little hand and said, "Sweetheart, Dad will take care of it."

We walked together (hand in hand) down the hallway, and we stopped at her door.

The door was shut. I got down on one knee and looked her in the eyes and said, "No matter what you hear, sweetie, don't open the door. Dad is going to kick his butt and throw him out of the window, never to return."

So I opened the door and walked into the room. I turned around and looked her in the eyes and said it again. "No matter what, don't open the door."

She just looked at me so scared and afraid. She just nodded at me okay.

I shut the door and made sure it latched. I started with the dresser. I took my arm and wiped it clean. Everything fell to the floor and made crashing sounds. In the deepest voice I could make, I yelled, "Get out!" I took her bed and flipped it over and kicked toys around the room. I tipped over the toy box. I made as much noise as I could. I trashed her room so bad. I opened her window and said, "Get out, and never come back!" I took out the screen and set it outside. I threw the blinds out the window and yelled, "Get out, and don't come back." It was a windy day, and the blinds were flapping in the wind. I walked over to the door and slowly opened it.

My little girl was standing there looking up with her little hands covering her eyes. I said, "He's gone and won't be back."

She slid one hand over so she could peek through her fingers. She slowly walked over to the door and pushed it open the best she could and slowly looked around. She said to me, "We had better get this cleaned up. Mommy is going to be mad."

I just started to laugh. We spent the next hour cleaning up the mess. I put the window back together and fixed up the blind. I fixed her bed and made it up for her. She sat on the bed looking at me. She said, "Daddy?"

I said, "Yes?"

She said, "I love you. Can we keep this a secret?"

I looked at her and said, "Okay, until you get older. It's kind of a funny story."

She said okay. That little girl slept great for the remainder of the time she spent there until we moved.

Over the next few weeks, I was not sure if I would make it much longer myself. I was feeling so sick. Every day I woke up, I was so grateful for another day. I still was getting up to take a shower before Leslie left for work every day. She would ask me every day if I was okay.

I would just smile and say, "I love you! Go to work. I will be okay."

I still had radiation appointments to get to. At times, I was living life right down to the very next second, it seemed like. I would be lying on the couch and snuggled up in Grandma's quilt, saying to myself that I could beat this. It's not my time yet, God. I love you, but not yet!

My CAT scan appointment came quickly. I was hoping that things would go smoothly. After the test, I had an appointment with the radiation doctor, Dr. Hart, and oncology doctor, Dr. Schwartz. I went in for an appointment with the radiation doctor first. Dr. Hart looked bothered when she came in.

I said, "How are you, Doc?"

She said, "I just was reading your results of the CAT scan, and it looks like the tumor did not respond to the two rounds of chemo or the radiation at all. In fact, your tumor has grown 2.5 centimeters one way and 3.1 centimeters another. It's so large, it has a dark area in the middle."

"What is it?" I asked.

She explained that it was a dead area of the tumor. As it grew, the core died out. "That's a very large tumor."

I was so blown away by the news. My wife, mom, and dad looked so defeated and hurt. I just smiled and said, "We will keep going forward with the treatment. I can take it."

Dr. Hart smiled and said, "Okay, James. I admire your courage."

I said in a soft voice, "Thank you, Doc. Try and have a good day."

We left and headed over to see the oncology doctor to basically hear the same news over again.

As I said earlier, Dr. Schwartz is confident and is well educated. This helped a lot when things were looking their worst. He came in the exam room and said hello.

He said, "I have looked at James's CAT scan, and it looks like the tumor has not responded to our treatment. In fact, it has grown a lot more than expected. James, how are you feeling?"

I said, "I am okay so far besides the side effects that we already talked about. I want to keep going with the treatments, Doc. After all, what else should I be doing?"

Dr. Schwartz smiled.

I said, "I can only think of one thing: fight for my life!"

Dr. Schwartz said, "I can't imagine anything but! Don't worry, James. We will beat this."

I smiled and said in a soft voice, "I am okay. I will see you for my third chemo appointment soon."

He said, "You guys have a good holiday, and I will see you later."

I said, "You too, Dr. Schwartz."

We left and headed home. It was extremely quiet in the car on the way home. We all walked in the house. I did realize what the doctors were saying about the tumor growing and growing fast. I needed some serious luck. I needed more than that; I needed a miracle!

Mom and Dad did not stay long. We said our goodbyes, and they headed home.

I looked at my beautiful wife and said, "I love you."

She started to cry so hard. I walked over to her and gave her a hug. As we were hugging, she said, "I love you too. I can't believe this is happening to us. It feels like a bad dream."

I thought to myself, It feels like this is the end of the road for me.

Later on that night, I decided to make peace with it and accepted what was coming my way: death. Once I accepted this, I decided to live my life one moment at a time from this day forward. If it had to be one minute at a time, then that's what it would be. After all, it was out of my control anyway. I had to get some sleep because it was back to the hospital in the morning for radiation. I accepted my destiny but was not giving up just yet.

When I woke up, I thought to myself, Sweet, I got one more day! I was going to make the best of it. My brother-in-law was coming to take me to radiation today. He came to get me, and we were on our way. We got to the hospital, and I told my brother-in-law to come in and hang out. After the little tour I gave him, they called me back for blood work. After the radiation treatment was over, I asked the doc for some stronger pain medication and some prescription-strength cough syrup.

I told her about the cough I had developed over the night. So she wrote me out the prescriptions, and we were on our way. My brother-in-law wanted to go to breakfast, so I decided to go with him. We were at Woody's in Walled Lake, eating. I felt so sick. I just sat there, watching out the window. The waitress came up to me and asked if everything was okay.

I said, "I just don't feel well! Thanks for asking."

My cell phone started to ring. I answered it.

"James, this is the nurse at the DMC Huron Valley Karmanos center. We need you to come back here right away. Your blood counts are dangerously low. Get here ASAP!"

I said, "Okay, see you soon."

I told my brother-in-law what was going on. We left to go back. He looked scared. He said, "You do look a little white."

I said, "Okay. It will be okay." The truth was I was freaked out! I kept saying to myself, "No, not yet!" I am not going to die today!

We got back there, and they took me back right away to the chemo room. It's a room filled with recliners.

There was like twelve to fifteen chairs all in a row. They said to have a seat. Dr. Hart was there waiting for me. She looked scared and asked if I was okay and how I was feeling.

I said, "I just feel tired, and I am on my pain meds, so I am not feeling much at all. God bless morphine." We all laughed a little bit. For some crazy reason it was funny.

She smiled and said, "Stay here."

The next thing I knew, they were hooking me up to an IV. She said, "You're going to be here awhile," and she explained about my blood count being dangerously low. "It's in the low hundreds."

I just smiled. I was clueless about what she was talking about.

"Thank God for trust," I said to my nurse.

She said, "I will be back to check on you soon."

After a while, I started to get hungry. I looked over at my brother-in-law and asked if he could get us some food, since we had to leave our breakfast behind at Woody's.

"Okay," he said, "what do you want?"

I said right away that Taco Bell sounded awesome!

He said, "Yes, it sounds good! I'm going."

So I gave him my order and asked the nurses if they wanted anything. They all said no.

He left to get the food, and the nurse came over to change my IV. About an hour later, my brother-in-law came back with the food. He said he had to go a long way to get the food. All the nurses were wishing he brought them back something because it smelled so good. Every time a doc, nurse, or another patient walked past, they would say something. After hours of IVs and repeated blood-count checks, I could go home.

It had been a long day, and I couldn't wait to get home to rest.

I thanked my brother-in-law for taking me and went into the house. My poor pups were so glad to see me, they about knocked me down. I said, "All right now, let's get outside."

I let the pups out, and I went in the living room to lie on the couch to rest. As I was lying there coughing, I coughed up a piece of something with blood on it. It made me finally feel that this could be the beginning of the end of my life.

As the holidays approached, I tried to see as much family as I could. I was telling them about the tumor growing, and it was not looking good for me. "Whatever happens," I said, "I thank you all for being there for me, and it's all going to be okay. I am pretty sick and coughing a lot. I am trying to get as much rest as I can." I spent a lot of time talking on the phone with family and friends. One of my friends from work had called to see how I was doing.

I explained to him that a few weeks ago, I got a call from our sick-bank committee person and that the sick bank had run out of funds. I said, "How can that be? I have been paying into the sick bank for twelve years now. I mean, Christmas is here, and I need that money to pay my bills. What the hell is going on over there?"

My friend said, "I don't know what to say other than I am sorry."

I said, "Can anything else go wrong?"

My friend was frustrated with this and wanted to look into it further.

I said, "They told me they restructured the way the sick bank is paid out."

He told me of the change they made back in July when we received our new contract.

I said I would have to wait until February 15 before the new funds were available. He said that there was nothing he could do. I said, "There is no sense in getting mad over it. It will not solve anything."

In the meantime, I had to file a motion with the friend of the court to let them know I was not working and of my condition. My friend felt bad for me and said to let him know if I needed anything. I told him I would and said good-bye. I thought to myself, On top of the cancer and side effects, I feel so sad and helpless. Talk about beating and kicking a guy when he is down!

As I lay there on the couch, wrapped up in Grandma's quilt, I said I wished to speak with God, and I said this couldn't wait. I said, "I don't know what I did to deserve this or why you're mad at me. I thought I was following your rules and was a good person, friend, husband, and father to my two girls. I can't die right now. My family needs me here. My daughters need me!

My wife needs me! God, are you listening to me?" I screamed at the top of my lungs, "GOD!"

I started to cough pretty badly. I spit up so much blood and debris. Once I settled down I drank some cough syrup. I got my composure back, and I lay there for a while, waiting for a response. Nothing came. I fell asleep and started to dream I was in a white room by myself, and I could hear someone talking. I remember saying, "Hello? Is someone there?" But no one responded. I just walked for a while, and I realized that I was pain-free. I had no cough. My hands did not hurt; my knees, ankles, and feet did not hurt. My back did not hurt anymore either. I thought that wherever I was, I liked being there. I felt safe and secure, like no harm could come to me. It was nice to feel perfect and pain-free again.

I had not felt this way in twenty years. I had forgotten what it was like to feel this way. Healthy! After a while of walking, I realized I was still alone and missed my wife and children. I said, "I have to go now. I'm not ready to stay here. Not yet." In a soft voice, I said, "God, are you listening to me? My family needs me more than ever."

I woke up from my dream. I felt confused and strange. I grabbed the remote to the TV and turned it on so I could see the clock. It was time for Leslie to come home.

Three hours had passed. I looked around the room, and the boys were lying down sleeping next to me. I looked up and Ally was staring down at me with one of her stuffed friends under her chin. I thought to myself, That was a strange dream. I got up to go to the bathroom. I was still in a lot of pain, and the coughing soon started back up. Leslie came home, and I began to tell her about my strange dream.

She just smiled. I never told another soul until I wrote this book. I said to Leslie that I couldn't say I had seen God. I could only say it was a dream, an extraordinary dream. I said it seemed so real.

She said, "I love you! Are you okay?"

I said yes.

"What do you want to eat?"

I said, "Pizza sounds good," so pizza it was.

We ordered delivery from a local favorite and feasted.

Christmas was here, and I had developed a heavy cough. I felt so sick and weak. I was lying on the couch in Grandma's old quilt. I just kept coughing and coughing. I drank some cough syrup doc ordered for me. I decided to take whatever I could because I had suffered enough pain. The day went by quickly, and Leslie made us a wonderful dinner. We stayed home for Christmas this year because of my illness.

I think the family was having a difficult time with my presence. I couldn't stop the coughing and spitting up blood. I just asked God to bless them and give them peace and strength to get through this difficult time. We had a great dinner, and I got the gift that I wanted the most, and that was to still be here and be with my wife on Christmas Day.

"I feel so blessed," I said to her.

We watched movies and made the best of the day as we could.

The next day, the coughing was intense with the debris and blood I was coughing up. The pain in my back and chest was so intense that I had to take more morphine that was prescribed to me. I was so miserable. I begged God to have mercy on me. I did not want to die! I was thinking I had just a few more days before my next round of chemo. I hoped I could make it through it.

The next day, I received a generous gift offer in the mail. It was an offer to participate in a medical study at Wayne State University. It appeared that my situation was unique, I guess, and it would help educate the medical students. The problem was I was so ill that I limited my travel, unless I absolutely had to go. So I declined the offer.

It was January now, and it was time for my third round of chemo. I still was coughing a lot and coughing up particles of bloody debris. I was so sick that I did not think I would live through the next chemo. I got up to go, and my friend Andrea was taking me this time. When she came to get me, she looked scared and worried. I told her, "Everything is going to be okay. Let's just do one hour at a time." I explained to her that the first day of chemo was eight hours long. She was okay with it. Leslie packed up some snacks and goodies to take along with us.

We got there and were called back right away. I introduced her to Penny and Melanie. I was bragging to Andrea about how I had my own private suite for the treatment (in a joking way). She just smiled until we got back there. She was impressed. I told her how lucky I felt to have caring nurses that understood. We sat down, and Karen came in. She asked how I was. I introduced Andrea to Karen. I asked Karen if I could have some water please when she came back. She said no problem.

I said, "My poor arms need some rest from all the poking from the needles."

They were black and blue from the top of my hands to my elbows. (I recommend a chemo port be installed before chemo starts or soon after.) My port was soon to be installed. I actually was looking forward to it. It was just weeks away.

Andrea and I talked all day, a little about everything. She asked me about having a benefit at the local club they belonged to. She said it would help a little since my sick-leave pay was canceled from my work. I gave it a little thought and then agreed to it. The medicated cough syrup started to kick in and was helping a little. I was telling Andrea about coughing up those particles. I said I couldn't help but think I was going to die.

I felt so sick and weak. I said I decided to take the pain medication because I was tired of suffering. Between the medicated cough syrup and morphine, I was doing okay. Then it hit me and hit me hard; I got quiet and thought about the patient in the lobby on my first visit here. I couldn't help my tears. My heart went out to that couple that sat there waiting. The women who sat there with him looked so scared and defeated. The man looked like he had had enough.

I realized that man probably felt the same way I felt right now. I just dried my tears. It was not like I had lost my will to fight, but this thought gave me inspiration to fight more and keep fighting. I did not want anyone to look at me that way ever. I thought to myself, I am going out kicking and screaming, just like I came in!

Andrea looked at me and did not say a word. She smiled at me. I just smiled back with an inspired look on my face. I never said anything about this to anyone, until now.

A few minutes passed, and Andrea said she prayed for me a lot. I was telling her about all the calls and cards of prayers I received from family and friends. May God bless you all! At the end of the chemo treatment, I said my good-byes to everyone, and we headed home. I thanked Andrea for her company and the ride. "I love you, Andrea! Thank you for being a good friend! Please don't cry!"

By the end of the third day, I felt pretty bad. I was back at home, lying on Grandma's quilt coughing and coughing up particles again. I could not eat and I could barely drink anything. I thought this was the end of me for sure. I was telling Leslie that I thought I was dying.

She kept saying, "Keep fighting! You can do it."

I thought to myself, You got to believe you can do it. I had lost about twenty-five pounds at this point, and I felt so weak. Later that night, I was lying in the tub sick as hell, thinking about all the great memories and special moments with my girls. They were so fun to be around. I really tried to be the best dad I could be. They are so loved. My youngest daughter was a little adventurer.

When she was young, she loved to go sledding. One winter when she was four years old, she asked me to make her a bigger sled hill. We had a small hill on the side of our property that they could sled on, but that became a beginner's hill in her eyes after a few runs.

She said, "Dad, do you think you could build me a bigger hill?"

I thought, No problem.

I got the shovel out and made the takeoff ramp two-feet high. After a couple runs, she said, "Dad, do think you can make it bigger?"

I thought to myself, All right, you babies! "Yes," I said, "I can make it bigger. However, you will need to go in the house for a while so Dad can build it. I will come and get you when I am done."

I walked over to the shed and fired up the plow tractor. I started pushing snow all the way to the top of the hill and made this giant pile to work from. I carved out a nice little path for the saucer sled to go in with the spade shovel. This hill had a launch drop of about five feet and then ran into a smooth path with sides. Then I went over and got the garden hose. I hooked it up to the outside faucet and sprinkled water over the whole thing.

You should have seen the eyes on this baby girl's face when she came out. She looked so excited. She climbed to the top with her sled on the steps I made. She set her sled down and climbed on. I gave her a little push and, swoosh, she was gone. She was going so fast that she cleared the landing ramp on this little jump I made halfway down the hill and sledded all the way over to the other side of the yard. She stood up after she stopped.

She looked at me with a huge smile and did not say a word. If I had to put it in words for her, she would have said, "Now, Dad, that's what I am talking about!"

She ran in the house to get her older sister to see the hill to play on. I just fell to my knees; I was so tired from building this thing. The dogs were out running around, so I sat out there for an hour with the pups and watched the girls have a great time.

These were some of my great memories with my girls. I had so much time to think. I decided to focus on all the great moments. Ones that made me smile at the most.

When I woke up Friday morning, I thought, Awesome, one more day!

I soon realized my coughing had gotten a little better, and my back pain was near gone. I was not sure what was happening to me. Leslie was up and getting ready for work. I said good morning to her and told Leslie how much better I felt and that the pain was near gone in my chest and back areas. She said she was happy for me.

She came over and gave me a big kiss and then looked at me and said, "Keep believing!"

She had to go to work. Dad came within a few minutes and took me to my radiation treatment. We slipped in and out without having to wait at all. We decided to go to Woody's again for breakfast.

I was telling Dad that my coughing had almost stopped and that the pain was near gone from my chest and back. He was surprised as much as I was. I said I finally had an appetite. It felt good to eat. Dad had a busy day planned, so he dropped me off at home. I went the rest of the weekend not having to take any of the heavy pain medications. This was nice for a change.

Monday came, and I had to go back to radiation for my last treatment. Dad picked me up and headed for the hospital. After the radiation treatment, they called us back to the exam room.

Dr. Hart came in the room. She asked me how the cough was doing. I said it had just about stopped Friday morning. I said the pain in my back and chest was not as bad.

She said, "Let's do another CAT scan and see what's going on in there."

After a few minutes, the doc came back with a cart and another doc and a technician.

She said, "They will take you down and have the CAT scan done and bring you back to me."

I said okay and climbed on the cart. It was the usual test. They hooked me up to an IV. I lay on a flat table, and I passed through a large ring that rotated inside. Just before I went in the large ring, they injected me with a medication and sent me through. That's it. When I got down to the CAT scan room, there was a patient ahead of me.

The technician said, "James, we are going to leave you right here for a minute or two. As soon as she's done, you will be next."

I said okay. Soon enough, I was in there. The test was done, and I was on my way back to the room. Dad and I waited around for a while. Dr. Hart came in with the news. She looked amazed.

She said, "James, your tumor has shrunk down a lot—to about half its size."

I said, "You are kidding me." I thought to myself these past three weeks that I was dying. I said, "We all thought I was dying, and it actually was doing the opposite. My mind was racing with all these thoughts. It's not that I lost my faith or hope or the will to live. It shrank! All of that coughing and pain! Oh my God. Thank you, God, for listening to me. That's awesome!"

Dr. Hart said, "I am so happy for you! By the looks of the scan, your pulmonary artery is exposed enough, and there is room to operate." She smiled.

I was so excited! I had so many things going through my mind, especially because of the last few weeks. I mean, they told me I had inoperable, stage-four lung cancer. I told myself to accept the good news already! All that pain I went through. It hurt so badly. I sat there thinking to myself.

We all thought the tumor was growing and getting bigger with all that coughing and coughing up debris. It was the total opposite. It was shrinking! All that pain I went through was the tumor tearing away from my chest cavity. Coughing up debris was because the tumor was dying off and breaking up. I was so excited that I could not wait to tell my wife and the rest of my family. It's a miracle! I thought. I said, "Thank you to God! Thank you!"

I said, "Thank you, Doc!"

She said, "You're welcome. James, that's really remarkable, and I am amazed. This is definitely something I don't see often." The tone in her voice changed to serious. "I mean, the odds were totally against you. Somebody is looking out for you, James."

I said, "I wish I could give them a big bear hug right now and say thank you to them." Just in case you're watching me now, I thank you with all of my heart! I owed someone a big bear hug. So I gave it to the doc.

She said, "Please don't get too excited because you still have a very serious surgery to get through."

I smiled at her and said, "The surgery is the easy part, Doc!"

Doc was smiling. I told her we would be in touch.

I said, "I have a surgeon to get a hold of."

She asked me to let her know when the surgery would be. I said I would call or stop by. Doc walked out, and we were on our way to deliver some great news.

I was so excited! Dad and I walked out to the car. I got back in the car and on the phone right away to tell my beautiful bride the good news! I felt so alive, although I was not entirely in the clear. But alive! I had called my brother, Jerry, to tell them the news. Dad was on the phone with Mom. We were headed home. Dad and I got back to my house. By the end of the night, I had a cauliflower ear or what felt like it; I guess from talking on the phone so much.

I had set up an appointment with the surgeon to go over the chemo port he was going to install. It was just within a few days. I told his nurse about the good news and asked her to let the surgeon know of it. The appointment came with the surgeon to talk about the chemo port. We also set up the appointment for my lung surgery. It was set up for the end of February. He asked me how I was doing.

I said, "I feel really good, and I am excited about the news."

He said, "I am happy for you, but you're not in the clear yet. Please understand how serious this surgery is."

"It's okay, Doc. I do understand what you are saying. Are you listening to me? I said it's okay. I will get through it with faith and hope."

He started to tell me about the procedure to remove the tumor.

I had to stop him because it was sounding pretty rough. I said, "Doc, I trust you! Please do not tell me any more. You want me to show up, don't you?" I shook his hand and said I would be there. "Let's get the port done first. We can talk some more then."

He said okay.

We all left and walked to the parking lot. Leslie had to go to work, and Mom and Dad had to take me home. I was excited to get the port because it would be the end to most of the needle pokes. I wish I had it installed right away when I was diagnosed. I regretted this pretty badly.

I was talking with Andrea, who was hosting the fundraiser benefit for me. I was in need of some money to pay my bills. She told me that they had posted an AD in the Oakland press about the benefit and explained the details and the date of the event. I was telling her that the surgery for the chemo port was scheduled for the following Tuesday. The benefit was on Friday, and I said I planned on going to it for an hour or so if I was feeling okay from the surgery.

I said it would be good to go just before the poker starts. I was telling her how Dad was saying how he wanted to play in the tournament. I was telling her that my brother wanted to play in it as well. We said our good-byes. Later on my brother-in-law came over to see how I was doing. He started talking about how he wanted to play in the benefit tournament as well. He was going on and on about how he was going to win the whole thing. This was nothing new to him to talk a little smack.

Tuesday came fast, and I was nervous about the surgery. Mom was taking me to the surgery to have the port installed. She came to get me, and we were on our way to the hospital. It was all over pretty fast, and I was back in recovery. I was talking with the recovery nurse. She said I was funny while under the anesthesia.

I said, "Oh God, please do not tell me." A couple of minutes later, I started telling her what a character I was this one time when I was put under anesthesia when I was getting my colonoscopy done. I was so nervous.

They called me back and handed me a plastic bag and a gown and said to strip down and put my clothes in the bag, put the robe on, and lie down on the bed. Soon after that, the nurse came back and started the IV. The anesthesia doctor came in, and I asked her to give me something to help with the anxiety I was experiencing. The doc agreed. After about thirty minutes of waiting, it was time to go back. Whatever they gave me, I was out of it.

This was what the nurse told my wife: I grabbed the anesthesia doctor's hand and held it tightly. I said, "This gastro doc is strange. He keeps eyeballing me." I pleaded with her not to let him hurt me. I said just before I went under, "Please don't let him spank my ass!" I was out.

The nurse came out to talk with my wife and said, "Your husband is doing great. He had us laughing so hard. He was so funny."

Leslie said, "Oh God, what did he do?"

She told her the story, and they laughed together.

Anyway, the surgery was over, and Mom and I were on our way back home to recuperate. I said, "Thank you for everything," to Mom. She had done so much for me, and I was very grateful.

Jerry and Ruth were coming down for the weekend to hang out. Friday had come, and it was time to go to the benefit. I got into my brother's car, and we headed over to the local club where it was being held. I was surprised when I got there to see some old friends show up that I had not seen in years. A lot of my ex-wife's family was there. Some of them I had not seen in a long time. They were all glad to see me, and I was glad to see them. I had a great relationship with my ex's family. I do miss them. They all have a special place in my heart. They were cheering me on to continue to fight. They all are great people. It was good to see all those old faces.

After walking around for an hour and talking with everyone, it was time for the poker tournament to start. I walked to the center of the room and said thank you to everyone and expressed how grateful and blessed I was to have friends and family. I wished them good luck and to look out for each other tonight.

Jerry, Ruth, and I headed home for me to rest. We watched some movies, and I finally went to bed. Leslie came home after cleaning up. I thanked her for everything she does. I know I said this already, but I honestly can say I have the best wife in the world. I would be so lost without her.

The next day, Andrea came over with some money from the benefit, and I just let go. My tears were flowing. I cleaned myself up and said thank you to her. Just in case you're reading this, I want to say thank you to them again for their support and friendship! I love you all!

THE SURGERY

It was time to meet with Dr. Apostolou, the surgeon, and talk about the surgery. We got there and were called back right away. Dr. Apostolou came in, and we said our hellos. He asked me to remove my shirt to look at the port to see how it was healing.

He said, "It looks good. Let's talk about the surgery, okay?"

I said okay.

"We will go through the side under your shoulder blade. We will cut through there and spread your ribs apart. There we will have access to the chest cavity and have a better view of everything. Let me remind you how big the tumor is and where it is. I reviewed the CAT scan, and it looks like I have enough room to clamp off the pulmonary artery. James, do you have any questions?"

I said, "No, sir. I feel good, and I am ready."

"Don't do any chemo until the surgery is over," he said, "and we will go from there."

"I have no arguments with that," I said.

Leslie, Dad, and Mom Dopke came with me to the appointment and were all very supportive. They all had a question or two about the surgery procedure, and the doc answered all of them. He said it was still scheduled for the end of February and reminded me of the risks.

I said, "I am okay, after all, what choice do I have, Doc?" I looked Doc in the eyes, and I said, "I have faith, hope, and confidence in you!"

"Thank you, James. You are a strong man, and I will see you in a couple weeks."

We said good-bye to him and left for lunch. I had all these thoughts going through my mind about the surgery but decided to keep them to myself. I found it best not to talk about it, or I probably would not have shown up for the surgery. There was no sense in worrying the family any more than they were already either. The next morning Leslie headed for work, and Mom, Dad, and I headed for breakfast. While we were eating breakfast at Woody's, we were talking about going ice fishing the weekend coming up. I thought it would be great to go up north and relax. So we decided to go up to Rose Lake. It was up by Jerry and Ruth's place. When Mom and Dad dropped me off at home, I started to pack my suitcase.

Friday came, and Dad and Larry came to pick me up. When we got up there, it was cold, quiet, and absolutely beautiful with all the snow. We stayed over at Larry's place that was close by Jerry's for the weekend. Larry fired up the wood stove so we could get some heat. We hung out at Larry's place most of the day on Friday. I watched all the deer going back and forth through the windows for a while. We played some poker for an hour or so, and then we went to the all-you-can-eat fish fry at the local bar.

It was not too bad. We finished up eating and went back to Larry's. For the rest of the night, we played some poker and had a few drinks. We got up the next morning and ate a little breakfast. Cherry Pop-Tarts! Yummy! We got dressed to go fishing. I had so many layers of clothes on, I could barely move. We got down to the lake, and it was so beautiful there. The snow was real deep and had covered the trees and pretty much everything else. Larry brought his 4x4 quad and gave Dad and me a ride down to the lake. We walked the rest of the way to the spot where the ice shanty was.

Larry started drilling some holes for Dad to fish out of. The ice was over one foot thick. We were feeling safe. My niece Jackie and my brother Jerry came down to fish with us. Jackie had a sweet ice shanty that my brother made for her. It was a comfortable seventy degrees in there with the heater, and it had plenty of room for three. I had so many clothes on that the only cold air I could feel was on my nose. I decided to stay outside and relax in a fold-up chair by Dad, Jerry, and Larry. I decided not to do any fishing at all. It just felt good to be there and relax and visit. I was trying to rest as much as I could. I called Leslie to let her know we were doing okay and that I missed her and the puppies.

I spent more time visiting Jerry and Jackie. It was good to see the family again. After a catch-less day, we headed back to Larry's place, and I asked Dad about going to eat at my favorite pizza place, Mineral Springs!

Dad said, "You sure love that place."

I said, "I sure do."

He agreed, and we left to go eat. Jerry and Ruth had met us up there. The pizza was fantastic. After a good night of visiting and hanging out, we headed back to Larry's place to rest. I grabbed the TV remote and turned on the satellite. I started flicking through the channels and found a classic movie to watch, Smoky and the Bandit! I love Jackie Gleason in that film. We watched that movie and headed to bed. At night, all you could hear was the firewood crackling. It was very peaceful there. I lay there with my wife's nightgown she packed for me and one of Ally's favorite toys to remember them by. I could smell her scent, and it gave me comfort. I snuggled up with them under my chin thinking about them as I went to sleep.

The weekend went fast, and we were heading home already. I really enjoyed my time with Leslie's dad and Larry. He's the father I never had growing up. I feel blessed to have him and Mom in my life.

They sure had helped me a lot with rides to and from the doctors' offices and a lot of advice and guidance. Dad dropped me off at home, and we said goodbye. I got a big greeting when I returned home. I was glad to see my wife and family. My puppies were jumping all over me. Chewie was trying to knock me down. I finally got them to calm down a little. I gave Leslie a big hug and a kiss. I then went and lay on the living room floor for a while with the puppies. They missed their daddy!

I was listening to my body and my heart. It was telling me to rest! I knew I could do no wrong if I did that. I spent a lot of time also talking with Leslie and the girls. I wanted them to know that if anything did happen to me, they were loved more than my life itself. I was glad to be back at home. I went in the bathroom and took a hot shower and cleaned myself up. I got out and was looking in the mirror. I said, "Bald is beautiful."

As I walked in the bedroom, Leslie whistled at me.

It was time to hit the sack. I tried to sleep and not think about the surgery. It was hard not to think about the stage-four lung cancer too. I was thinking about the odds of survival; I mean, 20 percent just sucked. I said a nice prayer, asking God to look after my wife and children and to help them heal their hearts if I did not make it through the surgery. I said thank you to God for everything so far in my life! I nodded off to sleep.

The two weeks had passed fast, and it was nice not being on chemo and radiation. I felt like I was getting a small piece of my life back. I was getting ready for the surgery and was feeling pretty nervous. I looked at the girls and asked if they were okay. They both said yes. They asked if I was.

I smiled and said, "I am. God's here today with me in my heart, and I will be okay."

They just smiled back. I asked Leslie if she was ready to go. She needed a few minutes to gather a few things. I said for her to take their time. A minute later she came out ready to go, and we were on our way to the hospital. When we got there and walked into registration, some of my family was already there to wish me good luck.

I said to everyone, "Please try not to feel bad, and please be strong for me. I love you all." I smiled at them.

Soon after signing in, they called me back. I stood up and said, "Good-bye for now," to everyone. I gave my wife a big hug and said, "I love you" to her, and I said, "I love you all, too."

I turned and walked away with the nurse. She introduced herself and asked me what I was here for today. I smiled and said, "I have a large tumor in my right lung, and they are going to remove it today, or at least try."

She smiled and said okay. She said, "This is your room, James. Please remove all of your clothes and put them in the plastic bag. Please put the robe on with the opening in the rear."

I smiled at her and said okay. The robe this time came with a pair of white panty hose. I thought, Oh hell, this can't be the way I spend my last day here. I just shook my head. I put them on and slid back in the bed. She explained why I had to wear them and said everyone had to. I said okay and left it at that. She installed the IV. The anesthesia doc and an assistant to the surgeon doc came in the room, and it seemed to make me laugh because of the last time. I explained a little bit, and the docs laughed.

We talked about the seriousness of the surgery and the chances of death. I said, "I am all right, and I realize the situation. The surgeon has explained it all to me weeks ago."

Doc said, "If you will, then write on the area to be operated on with this marker."

So I did. I wrote, "Right here please," with an "X" marking the spot. Then I put a big circle around it. I handed her back the marker. The anesthesia doc asked me about doing an epidural shot. It's a needle put in your spine to numb the surgery area to be operated on for a couple of days. I was concerned at first until she explained how much pain I would be in when I woke up, so I agreed to have it. I signed the papers and waited to be taken back.

After a few minutes alone, I started to cry, and tears were running down my face because the truth was, I did not want to die. And for some crazy reason, the reality of the situation seemed to come crashing in at this very moment. I thought to myself, Suck it up and dry your eyes, and be strong for your girls and your wife. I guess it's just impossible to control all of your emotions.

After about ten minutes, Leslie came back to wish me good luck and sat with me until they came to get me. The girls came back for a minute to say good luck and to say, "I love you, Dad."

I told them I would be okay, no matter what. I said, "I love you girls so much."

We hugged, and I said, "Stay strong for Dad now!"

Mom and Dad came back to say good luck to me, and the girls headed back to the waiting room.

Dad made a joke about my white tights. I smiled at him and said, "I am secure in my manhood—secure enough to wear these to breakfast at Woody's!"

We all laughed. Mom and Dad left, and it was time to go back. I said good-bye to my beautiful bride, hoping to see her again. The nurses did not say much on the way there. The surgeon was there waiting and smiled at me when I came in.

He said, "James, you stay strong for me." He started to go into detail on what he was going to do, but I stopped him.

"Doc," I said, "no matter what happens, just give me your best."

He smiled through the mask and turned to look at the anesthesia doc and said to go ahead and put me under. Doc said, "Could you count to five for me?"

I never even got to say a word. James, out!

I woke up in intensive care. I was looking around, and realized I was hooked up to all kinds of machines. I had this facemask on with hoses connected to it. It was pumping oxygen into me. My nose was sore from it, and it made my eyes water. As my first waking minute approached, the pain started to get intense. I started yelling for my wife to come, and no one was there. It hurt so badly that I felt like I could barely breathe.

The nurse came in and asked, "What's wrong, James?"

I told her, "I hurt so badly that I feel like I'm being tortured. What's wrong with me?"

She said the epidural shot must have not worked. "I will get you some pain medication, but I need to know the level of pain you're in."

I yelled, "Get the damn shot, or I will get it myself."

She said, "Hold on, James! I will be right back! Just hold on!"

She left to get the pain medication. After a couple of minutes of being tortured, I realized how hard it was to breathe. I felt so light-headed. My wife had come in, and I was so glad to see her. She was asking me what was wrong, and as I started to speak, the nurse came in with the pain medication.

As she was giving me the shot, she was explaining what was going on to Leslie. Leslie kept asking if I was okay. I said, "I am glad to be alive, and as soon as the pain meds start to work, we will go from there. Holy shit!"

She grabbed my hand, and she looked at me so scared.

I said, "Don't worry, Leslie, about a thing, because every little thing is going to be all right."

She smiled with tears in her eyes. I just stared at her, and I passed out. The pain meds kicked in.

I must have slept a long time. It felt like I missed a whole day. When I came to, I looked around the room, and Dad was snoozing in the chair close to the side of the bed. I reached over and tapped his knee with my foot to wake him. I couldn't talk too loud because my throat was sore, and I had the sleep apnea machine hooked to my face. I took off the mask and set it on the side of my bed.

I said, "Dad," in a short, raspy voice.

Dad woke up and said hello. He asked how I was doing. I said I was not sure yet because it hurt all over. I asked what day it was.

Dad said, "You've been sleeping for two days."

I couldn't believe it. I said, "How bad is it? Did they take my whole lung?"

Dad said, "No, they could keep just the lower lobe."

The nurse must have heard Dad talking and came in to see how I was doing. She asked how my pain level was.

I said, "It feels like I had my lung removed."

She smiled and asked me if I needed it increased. I said, "Just a little, please. I want to stay awake for a while. That stuff is powerful."

She made the adjustment and walked out. I asked Dad how Leslie was doing and how the girls were doing. Dad said, "Everyone is fine, and Leslie waited a long time for you to wake up but had to go back to work."

I said, "That's understandable." I said thanks to Dad for staying with me.

He smiled and said, "Of course. You're my son."

I smiled. After a couple of hours of talking and being awake, I tried sitting up; I had to go to the bathroom.

Dad said, "Number one?"

I said, "Dad, I have to go number two."

He was looking at me and said, "There is a bathroom back there. I don't know how you will get back there though. It's pretty tight."

I realized the room was really small, but it had a bathroom in it. So I said, "I got to go," and I started to unhook all the tubes and wires. Alarms started going off, and I was up and on the move. I made it to the restroom before the nurses and doctors came in.

Doctors and nurses came running in the room! They said to Dad, "Where is he?"

Dad pointed at the restroom.

The nurse said, "James, are you okay in there?"

I said real calmly, "I am now."

I cleaned myself up and washed my hands the best I could. I turned to open the door, and there were five people in there all staring at me.

The on-call doc said, "You gave us all a good scare."

I said, "Yes, how's that, Doc?"

He said, "You unhooked your heart monitors and oxygen monitors, James. That's where the alarms are hooked up. They are triggered to go off when your heart stops or your oxygen level gets low."

I said, "I'm sorry, Doc, but I had to go."

He stood there shaking his head back and forth and smiled. Doc turned to the nurses and asked if the pad was explained to me.

I interrupted him and said, "What pad?"

Dad said, "He just woke up a little while ago."

Doc said, "Get this cleaned up." As he got to the door, he said, "James, just stay in bed, please."

The nurses began to hook me all back up.

I said, "Okay, Doc." I felt bad about the nurses getting in trouble.

My assigned nurse said in a whisper, "Why didn't you call me?"

I said, "I didn't think it was a big deal. I realize this now, and I will stay in bed. If I have to go again, I will call you."

She said, "That's what this green pad is for."

I motioned at her to come closer. I said in a whisper, "I'm sorry, but I will not go on the green pad. I am totally capable of getting up and going. Please, can you take a couple of minutes and make it so I can reach the restroom without unhooking all these tubes and wires again, please?"

She said, "You're supposed to stay in bed. You heard the doc."

I said, "Yes. Yes I did."

She looked at me for a few seconds and said she would take care of it. She whispered, "You better not tell a soul."

I said I would keep it on the down low. I just smiled. For the record, I kept it a secret. She made the necessary adjustments and left the room. I looked over at Dad and said, "Nice going, Dad." I smiled at Dad.

We both started to laugh. Dad just looked at me with the "oh, son" look and shook his head back and forth.

The heart doctor came in the room and introduced himself and asked how I was feeling. I said, "I am confused here, Doc. What do I need a heart doctor for?"

He explained that during the surgery, my heart went into overdrive and was beating over two hundred beats per minute. This happens sometimes when the human body goes into shock from a major trauma or surgery. "You were one of the lucky ones, James."

I am not surprised with all the crazy luck I have been having, I thought to myself.

The heart doctor said, "I was here yesterday to check on you, but you were asleep."

I said thank you to him.

Anyway, he said, "You appear to be doing okay now, and I will come to see how you're doing in a day or two."

I said, "Okay, Doc. It was nice to meet you."

Later that day, Dad left, and Leslie came to visit. I missed her so much. I gave her the hug of a lifetime and started to tell her about my day. She already heard about the restroom incident on her way up from the nurse. Leslie laughed a little and said, "Try not to get in any more trouble."

I just laughed. I said, "That's something that seems to follow me. It's a little funny, babe. I love you!"

She finally gave in and gave me a smile. Leslie stayed as late as she could. We talked about the family for a while. I asked how the girls were. Leslie said real well. She looked so tired and stressed. I asked her to go home and get some rest and told her I would be on my best behavior, I promise. "I love you!"

We kissed, and she headed for home.

On her way out the door, I started to sing in my raspy voice, "Don't worry about a thing because every little thing is going to be all right!"

She looked back and smiled. That night they hooked me up to a sleep apnea machine to help me breathe and exercise the baby lung. I did not care for this thing at all. I could not sleep much at all anyway because every two hours, someone was coming in either to take vitals or blood sugar or a doc was checking up on me.

The next morning there was a shift change, and I was assigned a new nurse. I was doing a little better. The surgeon, Dr. Apostolou, came in to see how I was doing. He had heard about the bathroom incident and laughed with me. I said I was sorry. He started to tell me how strong of a person I was and that the surgery took a long time and had some complications. "Almost five hours in there," he said. He went on about my heart issues and how big the tumor was and said there was a lot of scar tissue. However, he felt they got the entire cancer tumor removed.

He said that I had just a small right lung now instead of no lung. He said, "I had to remove the upper and middle lobes."

"I'm okay with it," I said. "I'm glad to be alive. I thank you for that."

He said, "I can't take all the credit. If you were not a strong person, it wouldn't have worked. You gave us a little scare with your heart rate jumping up. However, everything worked out great in the end."

I said, "Thank you again, Doc."

He said he was here the day before to see how I was doing, but I was sleeping. I said that's okay, and thanks for checking up on me and for everything else. I shook his hand. Doc left, and the new nurse came.

He was a male nurse, and I could not help myself from giggling a little inside because of the movie Meet the Parents. The male nurse said they planned on moving me that day to a nice double suite on the next floor.

For a few seconds, I just stared at him eye to eye. I was thinking to myself, That is not going to work for me. I said to him in a firm but gentle voice with a hint of confidence, "Nurse! I am a private-room kind of guy.

He said, "What?"

I said, "I am saying that the double suite won't work for me. This is not The Bucket List where it's two beds to every room, no matter what! I know they have private suites here in this hospital."

He smiled and said, "I'm sorry, they're all taken."

I said real calmly, "Nurse, did you hear about my second day here?"

He said, "Yes, I did. We all got a great laugh out of it."

I said, "Look at it this way. I can be quiet in a private suite, or I can be the total opposite and be a real pain in the ass in a double suite. I am already in a lot of pain, and I find it easy to be really loud. However, if I was in my own room, I could change my focus."

He said, "I'll see what I can do."

I said, "Talk to my doc if you have to. Thank you, Nurse!"

A few hours had passed, and Mom and Dad came back to visit. I was telling them a little about my suite negotiation and hoped I got my point across without being mean or disrespectful to the guy. They both have had hospital stays and could understand. It is nice to have some privacy when you are that sick. About an hour passed, and the nurse came back with the suite update. I said hi to him and introduced Mom and Dad to him.

The nurse said, "It's nice to meet you both, and James, that suite situation is all set."

I said thank you to him very much and shook his hand. The nurse left the room, and Dad said, "How did you get a private room?"

I said to Dad, "I was thinking to myself that it was not going to work for me in a double room. I said to him in a firm but gentle voice with a hint of confidence, 'Nurse I am a private-room kind of guy. I am saying that the double suite won't work for me. This is not the The Bucket List where it's two beds to every room, no matter what.'" Mom and Dad laughed a little and then gave me the "oh son" look if you could imagine.

It was lunchtime, and I was still struggling with eating. I had to force myself to eat. However, I did it. I was sleepy after lunch, and Mom and Dad decided to leave so I could rest. I said good-bye to them and shortly nodded off. That night they transferred me to my private room. Not one word was said about it. It had its own bathroom, and that's all I cared about, and it had a shower too. As I was getting settled in my new room, I had more visitors that night from family. My brother, Mark, and his girlfriend, Tara, stopped by to visit.

We talked for a while about the surgery and how lucky I was to be alive. They all were impressed with my private suite and asked me how I managed to get such a room. I just said that this was all they had left and left it at that. Mark was remembering when he was in the hospital. He did not get the luxury of a private room. We talked some more, and they both wished me well and headed out.

It was your typical night in the hospital. The nurses came in like clockwork (every one-and-a-half hours). The morning had come, and I was still alive. I was hurting beyond what most people will ever endure in their lives, but I was happy to have a chance to fight to stay alive.

It was breakfast time, and I ordered the Hercules platter. At least, that's what I asked for. I actually was ready to eat. When breakfast came, the plate had a scrambled egg and one slice of toast and one tiny piece of sausage. I thought to myself, What the? I ate it and was still hungry. When the woman came back to pick up the plate, I asked if I was given the wrong plate. She said, "No, sir."

I said, "Could I have a menu, please?"

She said, "You didn't get one of those."

I said, "No, my nurse put in my order verbally." Then it occurred to me. I wondered if that male nurse was messing with me. I just smiled. Karma's a bitch, isn't it?

The surgeon's assistant doctor stopped in in order to give me a heads-up that they planned on taking out my drain tubes that afternoon and stated how painful it would be.

I said, "Just bring a shot with you, Doc. I mean your finest rum and something to bite down on will do."

He smiled and walked out. What I did not know was how much tape they used on my back. A few hours had passed, and Dr. Apostolou came back and shut the door.

He said, "Hi, James."

I said, "Hi, Doc."

He said, "My assistant came by to explain what to prepare for."

I said, "Hold up, Doc. He never said to prepare for anything. He said it would not hurt that bad. I said, 'Did you bring a shot of rum with you?' He said no."

Shaking his head no at the same time, Doc said it would be okay. "Go ahead and turn on your left side."

So I did.

He said, "Grab the bed rail."

So I did.

He said, "All in one motion now. Please bear with me." So he peeled back a little tape and began to pull the rest off. It hurt so bad that I yelled out.

"What the heck!" I said. "Doc, you're killing me here."

He said, "I told you it hurts. However, if you knew that it was that badly, you wouldn't have let me do it. It's important to be awake through this."

I said, "Oh, I'm awake!"

He asked if I was okay, and I said, "No pain, no gain, Doc!"

He smiled. Doc said, "Everything looks good. I'll come and check on you later. You get to rest now."

I said I would. I said, "Bring some strong rum with you next time."

He smiled. He turned to walk out. Just before he walked out the door, he said, "Very nice room, by the way," and he let the door shut.

I smiled. As I lay there with the TV off, staring out the window, I began to think how lucky I was to be alive. I started to think about life and achievements. I can honestly say I felt like the richest man in the world, not financially wealthy, but better than that. Having a great wife and kids, my family and friends, they are the best!

I nodded off to sleep and woke a few hours later to my finger being poked. It was the nurse taking my sugar level. I said good morning. My assigned nurse came in.

She said, "The physical therapy person is coming this morning to get you up and moving."

I said, "That's great that I need that. It's time to go home."

"Not quite yet, James," the nurse said. "I see your doctor came in in order to remove the drain tubes."

I said, "Yes, he did."

"It's still red, but it looks okay," she said. "Did it hurt?"

I said, "Not at all."

She started laughing a little. She smiled and left it at that. She probably heard me yelling from out in the hallway. She applied new bandages to the two wounds. Soon after the nurse left, my breakfast came. I ate half of it and lay back down for a while. I was not that hungry, for some reason. I was having trouble breathing and was looking forward to the therapy. I was hoping it would help me if I got up and walked for a little while.

My body had to get use to the massive change, and it was going to take a lot of time to adjust. The therapy person came in and introduced herself. She had me sit up, and she tied a large belt around my waist. She said, "We're going to walk awhile, and the belt gives me something to hold in case you fall or pass out. Hold on to this walker. Let's take our time, okay?"

I said okay, and we were up and walking.

She said, "This floor goes in a circle. Please don't walk by yourself, okay?"

I said okay.

She started to explain the changes that my body would be going through. "I'm sure you experienced how easy you get light-headed."

I said yes.

"That will take a long time to adjust. Your blood will start to store more oxygen, and it will slowly go away."

I asked, "How long will it take?"

She said, "Only time will tell. Everyone is different."

I said okay. I made it one lap around. She asked how I felt.

"Let's go one more time around," I said.

She asked, "Are you light-headed yet?"

"I am at the halfway mark on the first lap. If I don't push it, I will never get better."

"That's right. Do you think you can make it two laps?"

"I have to make it," and I kept walking. I was so light-headed, but I kept walking. I got back to my bed and said thank you to her.

She said, "Today was a great first day, and I will see you later this after noon. We will walk again."

I said, "That sounds great." I fell asleep or passed out. I'm not sure which, but I was tired. I slept for a while and woke up to the scent of my wife's hair. I said hi to her. She had climbed into my hospital bed and napped with me. She said that she missed me, and we hugged for a while. She said the puppies all missed me too. I said that I missed them. I asked her how she and the puppies were doing.

She said she was doing fine and couldn't wait for me to get home. I said by Wednesday night, I would be home. She said the docs were thinking at least ten days. I thought to myself, This is almost my fourth day here.

"Wednesday is my goal, sweetheart. I'll walk as much as my body will let me, and I will ask for weaker pain medication. I will make it." I loved the saying, "If you can dream it, you can do it!"

Shortly after Leslie left, my friend Larry stopped in order to visit. He was admiring my private suite.

He was telling me about the time he was in the hospital and was put in a double-occupancy room. I said, "I'm sorry, Larry, but all the rooms here are private." I was messing with him a little. He didn't buy into it at all. So I came clean and told him what was going on so far and how I acquired the room. He just shook his head and laughed.

He said, "Chemo makes you crazy."

Joking around, I said, "I have some here. I can pop a straw in it for you if you want to try it. Oh, Nurse, can you make my friend an X-20 chemo cocktail please?"

We both just laughed.

He said, "At least you still have your sense of humor."

I said, "I do, and I plan to go home Wednesday night if the doc will clear me."

Larry said, "That's a big goal. Try not to overdo it."

Larry said he had to get going, and I thanked him for stopping by. He said he would be in touch and left. Have you ever had a friend you can just think about, and they make you smile? That's Larry!

It was lunchtime, and I had ordered a chicken salad to eat and some fruit. The nurse came in for the blood-sugar test. As I finished up lunch, the physical therapy person came to take me for a walk. I was excited to be up and walking. It felt good to set a goal. I grabbed the walker and headed out. About halfway around, I started to get light-headed again. I just kept it to myself for now. She started to ask me questions about my cancer. I told her that they diagnosed me with stage-four, non-small cell carcinoma cancer.

She said, "You're kidding me."

I said in a short story that over the holidays the tumor started to shrink, and I could have the surgery.

She said, "That's absolutely a miracle. Good for you and your family, James."

I said thank you.

She asked how I was doing. I said I would like to keep going, and I came clean about being light-headed.

"Let's try three laps."

I said okay.

"James, if you can make it four laps, you would be okay to go home."

"That would be great. I would like to go home on Wednesday."

"That's a big goal," she said.

I asked her if she wanted to walk later if she had time, or if it was acceptable to walk with my wife. She said that would be okay because I seemed to be doing better. After three laps, I was pretty tired again and ready to sleep. We went back to the room, and I climbed in bed on my own this time. It felt good to make progress.

Leslie came back later, and we talked for a while. I was telling her what the therapy person said and that I would like to walk again tonight before she went home. Leslie said she was proud of me and to keep pushing to do better. I said that I was giving it my all and thank you. After dinner, we went for a walk. I said to

Leslie that I had to do at least three laps. So I grabbed a wheelchair in the hallway to hold on to. As we were walking, I said to Leslie how lucky I felt to be alive. I didn't know how to explain it, but somebody was looking out for me.

I just looked up to the ceiling and gave a wink. I said thank you again to God. She asked me about the pain level.

I said, "I am okay for now, and I am going to push it really hard tomorrow to take a weaker dose. I want to go home by Wednesday night. It gives me two days to push it as hard as I can."

She asked if there was something wrong with the hospital.

I said, "No, not at all. The room is nice, and all the staff is great. Even the food is okay. There is no place like home. I miss my wife and my family. I miss my bed and shower."

I couldn't wait to get home. After the three laps, I went back to my room and got some rest. Leslie stayed a little while longer, and then she decided to head home to get rest herself. As I sat there, I started to feel bad about all the hours my wife had to pick up because the sick bank at my work ran out of funds. I tried not to think about the lame excuses they gave me. I talked on the phone for a while with family and friends and then went to sleep.

The next morning, I got up to shower on my own. Next on the agenda was a good breakfast and a good walk. I asked for the weaker pain meds, and I got them. I was hurting pretty badly. However, I felt alive and eager to be independent. I felt more like myself not being so drugged up. Breakfast was delivered, and I went to work on it. The therapy person came up pretty fast as I was finishing breakfast.

I said, "Do you smoke?"

"Yes I do. How did you know?"

I said I could smell it on her.

She started telling me how she wanted to quit smoking and how hard it was.

"I know it's hard to quit because I am an ex-smoker."

"How did you quit?" she asked.

"I quit cold turkey. I just threw them out of the car window on my way home from work back in '97 and never smoked again."

She said she wished she could do that.

I said, "The secret to quitting is fighting one craving at a time. Every time you have a craving, find something to do until it passes. Just don't eat! Over time, the cravings get fewer and further apart until they're gone. It's really that easy if you do it one step at a time."

She said she would have to try it that way.

"You can do it. I did it for my kids and myself. Look at me now. I did not quit soon enough. Don't end up like me."

She smiled. It seemed to hit home for her. She did not say much the rest of our walk. I said, "Could we go for one more lap? I feel I can make it." I was so lightheaded already. After the fourth lap, we headed back to my room. I climbed in to bed and then said thank you to her.

She said, "I should be thanking you."

I just smiled at her and said, "Have a good day. I'll see you tonight."

My surgeon, Dr. Apostolou, came in order to check on me. He asked how I was doing with the lighter pain medication. I said I was doing okay. I told him I made it four laps this morning.

He said, "That's great. You just might make Wednesday."

I said, "I will do it, Doc. You'll see!"

He said, "I believe you will now. Have a good day, and get some sleep."

I said, "You too."

Doc left the room. I had some more visitors from family, and some flowers were delivered from Uncle Ed and Terry. They cheered up the room a lot and smelled nice. I visited with my brother Mark and Tara for a while. They decided to go because I was falling asleep on them. Later that afternoon, my mom and Jim stopped by to say hi and see how I was doing. We talked for an hour. They decided to go and wished me will.

I slept for about three hours and woke to the therapy person saying, "You're ready for a walk."

I said, "Give me a minute to wake up, and we will go."

I drank some juice and sat up all the way. I stretched out a little and stood up. I said, "You're ready."

She smiled and hooked the belt up. I grabbed the walker, and we started walking. She asked me about my life.

I said, "I am married to a wonderful woman, and I have two girls. I have three dogs at home, and all of them are missing their daddy." I told her about Chewie and all the issues we had with him. She laughed the whole time we walked.

I said I would like to walk behind a wheelchair, if that was okay. She grabbed a wheelchair for me, and we walked some more. I made it to five laps and seemed to be doing okay.

She was impressed and said, "I think you will be okay."

We went back to the room, and I sat in the chair. I said, "Thank you. I will see you in the morning."

She asked if I was going to be okay in the chair.

I said, "I think so."

She said good night and walked out. I stayed in the chair for a while and then went back to my bed.

My wife came back to see me just before bedtime. I was telling her about how I made it five laps, and tomorrow my target was six. She was proud of me. We talked for a while, and I listened to her vent for a while about her sisters. I thought to myself that I could write a book about them someday. I said to Leslie, "I love you very much! Please try to stay away from them for a while. We have a full plate of problems to get through as it is now."

She said okay, and we just lay together for a while, watching TV.

Wednesday came fast, and I was itching to go home. The therapy person came in for a walk. She hooked me up to the belt. We walked and talked some more. We got on the topic of second chances and what to do with it. I said, "The sky is the limit if you put your mind to anything you want to do and stick with whatever you try. You will fall sometimes. That's life. However, you will succeed if you never give up."

She said, "I believe that because of you. I mean, look at you and what you have been through. James, you are inspiring to all of us here at the hospital, and it truly shows you practice what you preach.

I said, "If you don't know this already, life is short. You have to appreciate every day God gives you. Make each day count as if it were your last day here. That's how I will live my life from this day forward."

She said, "What would you do after today?"

"First I have to heal up for a while. After that, I have dreams."

"What's that, if you don't mind me asking?"

"I want to make it back to work. That's first on my agenda."

"That's a very big goal."

"It's bigger than a goal—it's my dream!"

She smiled and said, "I believe you will make it."

We walked some more and on the fifth lap, I grabbed the wheelchair because I was getting light-headed, but I wanted to go some more. I said, "My next big dream is to inspire people with life-threatening illnesses and cancer to keep fighting. Life is so precious. I was thinking about writing a book? I want to visit people someday when my health is not threatened. Tell them my story and show them there is hope."

She said, "That's going to be easy for you. I mean, to look what you have been through, and you're here to tell the tale."

We walked around one more lap and went back to the room.

"That's six laps, James. Good for you."

I said thank you. She removed the belt, and I sat in the chair.

I said, "Dr. Apostolou is going to let me leave today."

She said she figured as much. I said thank you to her again for everything. She wished me good luck and said she was honored to meet me and left the room.

I got up from the chair and went to take a shower all by myself. I was on a mission. The nurse came in the room and scared the heck out of me when she asked if I was okay. I said I was fine. I got out and got dressed and climbed in to bed. It was a little difficult, but I was feeling proud. Dad had come to visit, and I was telling him I could go home today if the surgeon would clear me. I said he should be here shortly.

We waited for a while then decided to eat lunch. I ordered some food from the kitchen for Dad and me to snack on. The food came pretty fast. As we were eating lunch, Dr. Apostolou came in. We said hello to him. Doc said it was okay for me to go home. I was walking pretty well. I made it to six laps, the therapy person said! I seemed to be functioning on my own pretty good. My pain level was through the roof, but I was doing okay with it. I kept it to myself.

He said, "It will take a few minutes to process the discharge papers, and someone will come to get you to take you downstairs."

"Thanks for everything, Doc. I mean that from the bottom of my heart." I gave him a handshake.

"James, you follow up at my office in fourteen days, and we will look at taking those staples out."

I said okay to Doc and told him to have a good day.

He smiled and said, "Congratulations to you again on your survival."

I said thank you, and he left the room. About a half-hour later, the nurse came to pick me up to go. I was so excited to get home and be reunited with my family. Dad went to get the car. I climbed in, and we were on our way.

I got home in the driveway, and I could hear the puppies barking. They missed their daddy! Chewie, my biggest lab, makes sounds like Chewbacca from Star Wars when he gets excited. This is why I named him that. He was up on the window seat bitching at me through the glass. Dad and I laughed. The other two barked and barked. It was a wonderful greeting. I opened up the door and was attacked by the puppies. After a few minutes, the puppies all settled down.

The boys came over and climbed on the couch with me. We were all snuggled up on the couch and getting ready to watch a movie. It was western time again, and we were watching *Pale Rider*, another favorite western. Dad stayed for a while until the movie was over and just to make sure I was okay. Leslie came home from work early to see how her lucky charm was doing.

I missed her so much. I gave her the biggest hug I could give. She asked how I was doing. I told her that I was doing okay, in a lot of pain, but okay. She said that she picked up some bandages for my back.

I said, "That's great." I told the hospital that I did not want a home nurse. I said my wife had no problem changing the bandages. Doc said if we changed them every night, I should be fine. He said to give him a call if there were any concerns or issues. I knew we would be fine though.

I told Leslie of the nice greeting I got when I got home. I told her about Chewie bitching at me through the glass. It was pretty funny. I wish I could have video-recorded it. She laughed and rubbed his head and floppy ears. Leslie asked what I wanted for dinner. I said pizza sounded good. She said she figured. So we ordered our favorite local delivery.

It felt so awesome to be home. I lay there with my puppies after dinner, watching the TV. It was going to be a long recovery. I thought there was no better place than home because of my family and, of course, the comfy couch and bed and Grandma's quilt.

March was here already. I noticed the weather started to change. I was excited for summer. I was getting up every day with Leslie when she was going to work. I had to walk laps, even if it was in the house up and down the hall. I was alone through the day and did not want to push it too far. However, I still got some form of exercise in. I was doing okay. Every night we changed the bandages. My very good neighbor friends, Tom and Jill, looked after me as well. Tom came over and watched some movies with me from time to time.

Jill came over on Monday evenings to watch The Bachelor with Leslie and me. It was girlfriend night! What can I say? We had a lot of fun. Some Mondays, we had several female friends over. Jill made me dinners on occasion and was always looking out for me. I am very grateful to have good friends like these guys. They are irreplaceable! I just want them to know how much they are loved. I love you guys! Soon, the whole world will know!

Two weeks went by quick, and it was time to get the staples taken out. I was excited about this because as the wound healed, it tightened up the skin, and the staples started to hurt. We got to the surgeon's office and were called back. Dr. Apostolou came in and said hi to us.

He said, "Let's have a look at you," so I removed my shirt.

Doc pulled the bandages off to look at the drainhole scars.

He said, "They look very good. Another week of bandages, and they should be okay."

My wife said thank you.

Doc did not waste any time at all. He grabbed a pair of pliers and started to pull staples out. I could feel the relief as he pulled them out. Doc asked if it hurt, and I said no.

"No pain, no gain," he said and began to laugh at me a little.

I said, "That's right, Doc."

GETTING READY FOR CHEMO AGAIN

After he was done pulling all the staples out, he said everything looked great. He asked about my pain level. I said I was still doing okay. He asked how many rounds of chemo I had left to do.

"Three more to go."

He smiled. He said, "Please wait for three more weeks and then start chemo."

"Okay, I will set up the appointment."

"In the meantime, keep exercising and eating. Let's get that weight up. Go eat some fast food if you have to."

"Okay, Doc."

"You come back to see me in four weeks. Please call if there are any problems or concerns. You look great, James, and you're doing well."

I said thank you to him. We got up to leave. I stopped at the front desk to make my follow-up and headed home.

Over the next few weeks, I spent a lot of time visiting with my family and friends and doing a lot of exercising. I was up walking as much as I could. I would push it right to the point to where I would almost pass out. I was following my heart. It was telling me to go just a little further.

It was nice to see Josh and Julie and little Charlie, their new son. I was so happy for them. We spent some good times with these guys. They are great friends! We went to the Kenny Chesney concert at Ford Field in Detroit the previous year while I was having all those symptoms and swelling issues. My wife wanted to go so badly, and I just couldn't let her down. So I doctored myself up to make it through the night.

We had a great time with those guys. We had a nice visit while I was healing up from the surgery. We had some sliders from the best slider restaurant in the world: Bate's Burgers! Josh and Julie were very kind enough to bring some over. These guys are lucky enough to live close by to Bate's. I would be eating there every day if I could. Leslie and I both love this place.

As the weather got warmer, I went on a few trips to Walmart with Leslie. She bought me a nice outdoor recliner to lie in while I healed up. I couldn't wait to use it. I thought it would be great for the fire pit because I loved being outdoors. I demonstrated the chair at the store. This chair is sweet. It's like having a full recliner outdoors. Over the next week, I spent some time outdoors walking and hanging out with my neighbors and friends.

The chemo appointment was coming fast, and I was dreading going back. Over Christmas, Leslie had put up a window display in the kitchen area. The display read in red gel letters the word "Believe." It's been left up since Christmas. I see this every day, and it reminds of what's really important in life!

Since I was diagnosed, I have been able to look at my life from the outside looking in. Don't get me wrong, my life is not bad at all. However, it gave me the ability to live life one day at a time and to appreciate the little things that are really important. My life! I had put my life on hold and lived for everyone else for years. I had quit doing the things I loved to do, and this was soon to change. I thought, When I get healed up and make it back to work, I am going to start doing more things that I like to do.

You are only here one time. You should enjoy it! For me, having hobbies is important. More importantly, they are your loves! You have to enjoy what you do. I like being by the ocean and smelling the salty air. It's very relaxing for me. I like to write but was afraid what people might think so I never did it, until now. I love fast Mustangs and exceeding the posted speed limit—on the expressways only! Shhh! Don't tell anyone!

It was the end of March and time for the chemo appointment. I was doing well with my new outlook. I knew what was coming my way, but I was going to fight and fight some more. I wanted my life back. Mom, Dad, and I arrived and said hello to Penny. Melanie called me back. She took my vitals. She finished up and then took us back to my private suite. We said hello to Karen, and we talked for a while. They were all glad to see me doing well. I was glad to see them doing well too.

Karen hooked me up and drew some blood. The results came back, and we got the green light to go ahead with the chemo. As the day passed, I was already starting to feel sick. Eight hours of chemo is a long day. Karen came back in order to check on me. She said that I looked very well. She asked to see my scar, so I turned to show her.

Karen said, "It looks like it healed up great."

I said, "It was nice to have the staples removed. Those hurt pretty badly. The surgery was tough, and my chest hurts pretty badly too. Overall, I am feeling really good."

She asked me if I remembered to take the nausea medication. I said yes. I told her Leslie said hello.

The last chemo bag ran empty. It was time to head home. I said thank you to Karen, Melanie, and Penny, and we headed home. We made it back to the house. I thanked Dad and Mom for taking me, and they headed home.

The puppies were glad to see me and were climbing all over me. I pushed the boys off the couch and put Ally on the top cushion. I turned the TV on for some noise and fell asleep. I woke a few hours later feeling extremely nauseated. I got up to take some pills and came back into the living room and sat in the big chair for a while. Leslie came home, and we talked about her day. I said my day was about the same and left it at that. I passed on dinner and went back to lie down on the couch. A few hours later, I found myself back in the bathroom. I was feeling so sick. I got in the shower to get warm. I slid down and let the warm water run on me.

I was trying to think of something positive when I remembered my Mustang GT convertible in the garage. I barely had driven it this year. I started to think about my first day with it. I was so excited to get it. The car was white with a white top and had black leather interior. It had a V8 engine and a five-speed transmission. It was in October a couple of years ago, and we were having a great Indian summer. Leslie and I put the top down and headed out for some fun. When we got on the expressway, I cranked it up a little to 90 mph.

"This thing handles like a dream," I said to Leslie. "Do you want to drive it?"

Leslie shook her head no. "I just like to ride," she said.

"That's silly, babe. Come on." I started to pull over.

"No, I don't want to. I can't drive a stick shift."

"That's okay. I will teach you."

"No, I really don't want to learn."

"Really?" I said,

She said, "Really!" She smiled and with a sincere voice said, "I really like riding with you."

I smiled at her and said, "Do you remember that one time coming home from up north in the old Mustang?"

She smiled and said, "How can I forget?"

We had a 1989 Mustang GT convertible that was a little modified. This car had the loud pipes on it. On our way home from up north, we were going pretty fast. The car stalled. I looked down at the odometer to check the miles we drove. It read 181 on the odometer.

I thought to myself, That's odd. I usually get 185 out of a tank. The gas gauge was broken.

We were slowing down pretty quickly, so I shifted the car into neutral. We were coasting when I looked over at Leslie. That poor woman looked so frustrated. I grabbed her knee and shook it. She turned to look at me. I smiled at her and said, "It's going to be okay. When the car slows to 60, the rest of the gas will go to the pump area in the tank. It's the lowest spot in the tank. The car will start and get us a few more miles."

Leslie just looked at me.

I smiled, and I said, "You will see."

The car soon hit 60 mph, and I said, "Here we go." I turned the key over, and it fired right up. I put the shifter into the drive position and let her go. We passed a sign about a mile back that read: "Gas: 4 miles." I just was taking it easy for two miles until the hill approached. The car stalled again. We were back to coasting. Leslie just shook her head. I said right away that everything would be fine. We coasted all the way up to the hill and onto the exit ramp. We had the gas station in our sights.

We had to stop at an approaching stop sign. It was too risky to run and keep coasting. So I stopped! I looked both ways and smiled at Leslie. She didn't smile back at first until I turned the key over to start the car. The engine started, and I stepped on it to get going. We got over the bridge, and the car stalled again. I looked over at Leslie, and she still was not smiling. We coasted all the way into the gas station and came to a stop right in front of the gas pump. I turned to look at Leslie and said, "See, it was destiny!"

She finally smiled back at me. Her smiles to me are priceless! I could not help myself though when I said this as I approached the pump: "Out of gas? What the—?"

I turned back at Leslie as she sat in the car shaking her head at me. "Not funny," she said.

"Isn't it fun to fly by the seat of your pants a little?"

"No!"

I swiped my credit card and filled it up. I climbed in and started the car, and we were on our way. I said, "I love you!"

She smiled and said, "I love you too!"

Anyway, we were enjoying the newer Mustang we purchased. We drove it out to Mom and Dad's to show them the new car. They were happy for us.

We left from there and went driving another hour and headed home. I still have that Mustang and enjoy looking at it every day. Being so sick, I have not been able to drive it often. I do miss the old 'Stang from time to time. I think it was fun to fix it up and drive it daily and enjoy it. I see so many people put these cars they fix up in a garage and just stare at them. I personally do not see the fun in that! Get those keys out and go! That's what full-coverage insurance is for. I said it once before: Thinking of great moments that make you smile are very important to healing to me.

I got through the rest of the night and was up with Leslie in the morning, getting ready to go to chemo. This time my sister, Kristie, was taking me. She came to pick me up, and we were on our way. We got there, and I showed her around Dr. Schwartz's office. Kristie said it was very nice. She liked how comfortable it was there. I said I liked it a lot too.

I said, "Dr. Schwartz is great. He truly is one of a kind!"

Kristi said, "That's saying a lot, coming from you."

I smiled at her. I guess sometimes I can be a little abrasive. I said, "They offer you all the treats you want and drinks you can drink." I pointed out the fridge in the lobby. I said, "At this point, these guys have become an extension of my family."

I introduced her to everyone and went back to my room. I was bragging to her how I had my very own, private suite.

"That's too funny that you have your own private suite," she said. "How did you pull this off?"

Karen overheard her and stepped in for me. She said, "James is special and requires some special treatment. After all, he is here for three days in a row and needs to be as comfortable as possible."

She winked and smiled at me and walked away. I just went with it and smiled back. I looked over at Kristie and gave her a big raspberry. These are a must when someone deserves one. I reached over and grabbed the TV and pulled it over to me to turn it on for some noise. We spent the day talking about our family and other issues at hand. I said that we couldn't worry about things that were out of our control no more.

I said, "Look at me, for example. Can you put yourself in my shoes?"

She said, "No, I cannot. I can't even imagine what you are feeling or going through. How do you do it? What was it like?"

I did not get to talk with her much about what I experienced over Christmas and the surgery. I said, "Faith and hope got me through it. I was scared at first. I did not want to die. Then I was mad for a few days because I still did not want to die. Then I realized it was out of my hands now. It was out of my control. Although it was out of my control, I was not giving up. I did not think I deserved this, that's for sure. I had a few moments to speak my mind to God over the holidays. I said what was on my mind and spoke the truth. I asked God what I did do to deserve this hell on earth. I asked if it was something my father did, and I was being punished for it. I said I was sorry to God, and I repented all of my sins and my father's, if I can do that.

"I begged God, 'Please, God. Please listen to me.' I got no answer, and I started to cry. I prayed a lot and yelled at God a few more times. I figured if I was dying, I was going out the same way I came in! The last great act of defiance! Christmas was coming at the time, and I started to get real sick and thought it was the end for me."

She said, "I remember."

I said, "After a couple of weeks, I started to feel a little better, like I had a little more energy and coughed up a lot of the tumor. That's when I realized that God was listening to me, and my life was in his hands. I felt this warmth in my heart like never before. So now I don't worry anymore. I am not afraid no more. I wish the rest of the family could feel like I do right now."

Kristie said, "And how is that?"

"At peace! Doc and many others think it was a miracle for me to survive this. Either way, I am so glad to be here still." I looked up at the ceiling and said, "Thank you, God, for another day. I love you!"

My sister sat there and smiled. She realized that she was very fortunate to still have her brother there to talk to. We talked about hope and faith some more and how important it is and that it should be a part of everyone's life.

If you are reading this, live each day as if it were your last one. Make those moments count! By the way, you cannot take money with you when you die. Put it to good use, like donating it to cancer facilities that search for the cure for cancer. Help people that do not have insurance or cannot afford it. It would give them a little hope to live another day. I think God would give you that warmth I feel! It's priceless!

It was time to go. While I was getting my shirt on, I asked my sister if she wanted to go eat. We decided to get some breakfast. I said, "There is a restaurant by here that is awesome for eggs Benedict. So we headed there to eat.

She took me home after breakfast. I thanked her for taking me. I enjoyed my day with my little sister. I love you, Kristie! I went into the house to get more rest. I still had another day of chemo to get through. I was lying there watching a movie when my neighbor Tom came over to see how I was doing. We were just hanging out. Tom asked how I was feeling, and I just said about the same. It seemed like the appropriate thing to say instead of the truth; I felt like total garbage!

We watched the western channel for a while and talked about sports. Other than being sick, it felt like a great day of friends hanging out. Tom headed home for dinner, and soon after he left, my beautiful wife brought home our dinner, my favorite. It was just about the only thing I could eat during the chemo treatment. Leslie and I talked about her day. After a while of listening to my beautiful wife speak, she asked how my day went. I said,"My day was okay. Kristie and I had a good day talking. Tom came over, and we just hung out watching the western channel. It was a nice day. I really am dreading the next day of chemo."

We went downstairs to watch some more soaps that Leslie recorded for us. More General Hospital! A few hours had passed, and the itching began. That was the sign that my hair was going to fall out. I just started enjoying what had grown back so far. I kept that to myself. There was no sense in stressing my wife out any more than she already was.

I said to Leslie, "I am going upstairs to take a shower."

"Okay, I will be up soon," she said.

I went upstairs and grabbed a towel. I was itching so badly all over. I turned the shower on and climbed in. The hot water seemed to help a little with the itching, and it also washed the hair that fell out away. I must have been in there awhile because the water ran cold. I climbed out and got dressed.

I went into the living room to lie on the couch in the quilt for a while. Leslie came upstairs shortly after. She asked if I was doing okay. I said, "I am. I need to take the nausea medication."

Leslie grabbed it for me.

I was feeling cold and asked her to grab the heating pad for me. I got up to go to bed. I cranked that pad up to hot. I was so cold. I fell asleep for a couple of hours and woke up to a soaked bed because I was sweating so badly. I woke Leslie to tell her about the bed.

"I am going back into the shower. I will change the bedding when I get out of the shower."

I felt so badly that she already took such good care of me. Leslie got up and changed all the bedding while I was in the shower. She said, "Don't worry, it's okay!" When she got over to my side, she said, "Wow, babe, that's a lot of sweat. Even your pillows are soaked."

I felt bad for her having to take care of me like I was an infant. I kept telling her I was sorry.

Leslie said, "It's okay, honey. Don't worry about a thing, because every little thing is going to be all right." She was singing to me.

I smiled and sank down into the tub. I quickly started to think of something funny to take my mind off of things. I smiled as I remembered the time my wife and I went to my sister's for New Year's Eve. Leslie looked so gorgeous in her black dress. All I could say to keep it clean here for the kids is, "Hubba! Hubba!" She was stunning! Kids, take my advice here. "Do not let the beautiful ones fool you." She had a planned agenda that evening. When we got there we took some of that

Silver Star confetti and put large piles on each of the ceiling fan blades.

We used two whole boxes of it in the dining area alone. No one noticed us, and the fans went unused that night. A short time later the weather was much warmer and my sister and her entire family were sitting down at the table eating a large breakfast together. My brother-in-law said, "Could someone turn on the ceiling fan please?" My sister yelled, "I got it," as she walked back into the room with the final plate of food to serve. As the blades began to pick up speed the confetti began to blow around the room.

My sister and her family started to laugh because of the large amounts of it. She said what was funny was the endless supply of confetti. It just kept coming down. They scrambled to cover their food. My brother-in-law sat there trying to eat and finally said, "Enough already!" He started to get frustrated. My sister found it to be extremely humorous and laughed with the rest of the family until the last piece came softly down onto the table. As the last piece touched down she expressed that it had to be Leslie and I that had done it to the family. She told me that she felt like she was in a magical snow globe for five minutes. She loved it until it was time to clean it up. I loved the way she told me the story. It had so much humor to it.

Sorry, sis! I love you and hope that moment sticks with you forever.

I think of this moment often. When I was in my early thirties, we bought a female Jack Russell puppy and named her Josie. When she was a couple of years old we decided to share the puppy experience with the girls. They were so excited when they were born. The looks on their faces were priceless. We decided to name all the puppies after Disney Characters until they went to their new homes.

The girls really enjoyed playing with them as they grew. But it soon came time for them to go. Most of the puppies went quickly except for "Mickey." Mickey was special. For some reason he did not like anyone else. I told myself no one is taking him unless he says it's okay. Trust me when I say I stuck with it. I turned down several people when they came to meet him. Mickey was a boy, and every time someone came to take him he would growl at them and scare them away. It did not take long at all before I started to treat him as part of the family. I knew I could not keep him, so I continued to run the AD in the local paper. I thought I was stuck with him forever until this one day. A woman had called and told me of her five-year-old daughter and how badly she wanted a Jack Russell puppy.

I scheduled a time with the woman and explained the growling situation to her and said, "Let's see how they do together." She agreed. Saturday came and they pulled into the driveway. I walked out front to meet them and began to explain to the little girl that Mickey is a special boy and requires a lot of love. With a lot of confidence she said, "It will be all right, mister." I smiled and said, "All right, let's go meet him." I walked through the gate and opened the back door. I called for Mickey, and he came running outside. The little girl's face lit up with joy as she watched Mickey run around the yard.

I said to the little girl, "He knows a few commands already. If you say the word 'come' and point down to the ground in front of you like this, he will come and sit in front of you. He won't move until you do another command. Do you understand?"

She nodded yes. I looked up at mom and said, "This will be the test."

The mom smiled and said, "Let's see what happens."

The little girl watched Mickey run around the yard some more. He ran up the slide and lay in the girl's play fort. He peeked through the wood beams, staring down at the little girl as she approached the fort structure. She looked up at him and started up the ladder.

Once she got to the top Mickey slid down the slide on his butt. She giggled and laughed at him as he ran around the yard. The mom said, "That was so adorable."

I said, "Mickey is pretty funny to be around. He is like a little kid."

About half an hour had passed, and the little girl walked up to her mom and said, "I love him and I want him."

The mom said, "Let's see if he listens first like the man said."

I smiled at her and said, "Try and call him."

The little girl walked to the middle of the yard and yelled "Mickey!" He stopped in his tracks and looked at her.

She yelled, "Come," and pointed down to the ground in front of her. Without a pause, Mickey ran to her and stopped right in front of her. He stared at her in the eyes, and she stared back at him with no fear. I looked at the mom. She had tears in her eyes, and they had begun to run down her face. We both watched as the little girl leaned forward and whispered something to him. I watched as Mickey leaned forward and kissed the little girl on the mouth. I was amazed!

Here my "growling puppy" was won over by a five-year-old.

I said, "He is yours if you want him."

That was incredible. I was amazed my little boy just found a home. The mom cried some more and said, "She will take him. That was so precious."

She dried her eyes and asked if she could wait a few more minutes to be sure. I said, "Of course, take all the time you need."

I walked to the patio and sat down. They all played with each other for a while. Mickey was doing great interacting with them. The mom said, "He is so adorable." I explained the rest of his training to her. As they went to leave I said, "Could I have a second with Mickey?"

The mom said, "Sure, of course."

I knelt down and called Mickey over. He ran over and sat in front of me. I looked at him and said, "Dad is going to miss you, buddy." I rubbed the top of his head and said, "Be a good boy for them, okay."

Mickey kissed my face and ran back to the little girl. The mom said, "Thank you!" The little girl said, "I will take good care of him. He can sleep with me and share my toys. Thank you, mister."

I said, "You are welcome."

They walked through the gate together. Mickey followed right along as if it were destiny. They climbed into there van and drove away. I waved good-bye to them. I sat there thinking about that and other funny moments with family until the water ran cold again. I climbed out and got dressed and went back to bed.

I thanked Leslie for everything she did for me, and gave her a big kiss and a hug. We slept a little while, and soon the alarm went off for Leslie to go to work. I got up with her and went to sit in the chair. She packed her lunch and grabbed her bags. She gave me a kiss and said she would call soon to see how I was doing. I asked her to be careful and to have a good day at work. Mom was coming to pick me up for chemo today.

I got up to go get dressed. Mom came to get me, and we were on are way. I was telling her I wanted to take her to a new place for breakfast. I said they had the best eggs Benedict around. She said okay.

We got to Dr. Schwartz's office, and Penny sent us right back to the suite. I said good morning to Karen. She said good morning back. I had to do more blood work first to make sure my count was safe. The results came back okay.

I asked Mom how Dad was doing. She said he was tired too and feeling a little rough. I felt bad for him. She asked how I was doing. I started to tell Mom about my night.

I said, "The itching is back, and I started to lose a lot of hair already."

Mom frowned a little. I knew she felt bad for me.

"I was feeling pretty rough myself," I said. "As bad as I feel, I still have that warmth inside of me. I will get through this. Staying focused with a positive outlook is very important to survive."

I was telling Mom about some other patients that I had spoken with about cancer. They wondered, "When do you call it quits?"

I said to the man, "This is not tough for me to answer."

That man looked at me like I was nuts! I said to the gentleman, "Never! Never give up!"

He said, "But I have stage-three lung cancer, and I don't want to go through the surgery."

I smiled at the man and said, "Sir, the surgery was the easy part for me. You made it this far. You can do it." The man still looked confused. I said, "Do you like to be alive?"

He said, "Absolutely, I love life."

I said, "Then you keep fighting until you cannot fight no more. Did you know that I had stage-four lung cancer that was inoperable?"

The man said, "No, I did not know."

I smiled at him, looked him in the eyes, and said, "I understand how you feel. You are not alone here. Just don't quit fighting for your life."

I said to Mom that he smiled back at me and turned to his wife for comfort. I got up to go, and that man's wife looked at me and mouthed with her lips, "Thank you." I smiled at her and just nodded my head. Mom smiled at me. Karen came in to see how I was doing. She checked the chemo bags and went on her way.

Mom asked me where the breakfast place was. I told her it was real close by. We talked about Dad and how he was doing. Dad had colon cancer, and he was doing really well. His entire test came back positive, and he was done with chemo.

I was so happy for him. After a few hours of talking, the last chemo bag ran empty, and it was time to go. I said my good-byes to the staff and headed to breakfast. We got there, and Mom just loved the place; she enjoyed the eggs Benedict and atmosphere it gave. We talked some more about my future and what was in store for me.

I said to Mom, "At this point, I can only live my life one day at a time and enjoy each day as it was my last. So I do. I am okay with it. I used to be that person with a plan A and a plan B. So it was an adjustment is all. I really just am going to take it one step at a time. First, it is to get through chemo. Then get some strength back. One of my doctors does not think I can make it back to my line of work. He thinks I will have to do something else. He does not think I will have the integrity or stamina to perform my duties. I thought I would show them how much integrity I have and how much one full lung and a baby lung would do."

Mom laughed at me for calling my little lung my "baby lung." I am saying it again: "If you can dream it, you can do it!"

Mom paid the bill, and we were on our way home. I said, "Thanks for everything, Mom!"

She dropped me off, and I went into the house to greet the puppies. We all snuggled up again on the couch and took a nap. I slept a long time. I woke up later to Leslie coming home. I couldn't believe I slept that long. I woke up soaking wet from sweating. It was all the heat from the dogs and a fever that started. I gave Leslie a kiss and went into the shower. I stayed in the shower until the hot ran cold. I climbed out, got dressed, and went to bed.

I said, "I love you," to Leslie and started to wonder how she was handling everything. I asked, "How are you handling everything?" She said she was doing fine and that she was worried about me. I said I would be okay. She came in the room and laid with me awhile. It did not take long for me to fall back to sleep. I woke up in the middle of the night itching like crazy. I thought, Not again. Leslie got me an anti-itching stick that had a roll ball on the end. It was easy to hold onto because of the neuropathy problem. I used it a lot. It worked for a while at least to help me sleep.

I had the chills real bad again, so I was back in the shower to get warm. I got out and took more Tylenol to help with the fever. I started to feel a little better when Leslie's alarm went off for her to get up for work. She asked where I was. When I peeked my head through the door, I said good morning. She asked if I was okay. I said I was. "I just had the chills again."

She said she was sorry.

"It's not your fault, sweetheart!"

I offered to make her some breakfast, but she passed on it. Leslie got ready for work.

I told her I loved her and to have a good day. She told me to rest and to try and relax, but I wanted to walk for a while. I threw on some shoes and walked outside into the yard. It was getting warmer, and I could not be in a better place. I love our home a lot. It's like a northern setting in the backyard, with a lot of trees and shade. There were a lot of leaves on the ground, and it's pretty private. I poked around the yard, picking up fallen tree limbs, and decided to light a campfire in the pit.

I had some fire starter logs. I got the log and gathered up some more fallen tree limbs and lit the fire. I went to grab my new recliner chair and set it up. By the time I got that setup, I was ready for a nap again. I sat in the chair, and the thing reclined pretty easily. I was in heaven. I thought, If only my wonderful wife was here. I decided to call her at work and say hi and see how she was doing. When she picked up the line, I whistled that sexy whistle to her.

I said, "Do you want to play hooky?"

"Oh, sweetheart," she said, "you know I can't. You know I wish I could be there with you."

I said, "I know. It's okay. Are you doing all right?"

"I'm doing fine. Just really busy," she said.

"All right, I will talk with you later. I love you!"

"I love you too!"

I did not forget about my work telling me that they ran out of sick-bank funds or whatever excuse they used. Either way, I was not getting paid. Leslie had to pick up the slack. Hey, it is out of my control, I thought, and I am going to practice what I preach! I am not going to get mad or sad!

Hell, I am glad to be alive! I thought to myself. If we lose the house and the car, life is not so bad living in an apartment or with relatives. Starting over sometimes puts things in perspective and is a good, enlightening experience on what's really important: health, family, and friends! You cannot put a price on good health! I would trade any material thing for that, even my baby, my Mustang!

Over the next few weeks, I got to enjoy some great weather. I knocked out a few follow-up appointments and spent a little time with my youngest daughter. When she was around, I tried not to complain and stayed as strong as I could. She was very supportive about it.

When all of my hair fell out, she said, "Dad, you're even better looking than Bruce Willis!"

I smiled, and I said, "Thank you! Bruce is a pretty handsome guy, and that's a hell of a compliment. Maybe I will be in the movies someday?"

My daughter said, "I doubt it, Dad."

I said, "You never know!"

She just smiled. I thought to myself, Those babies!

It was a Sunday, and I had to take her home; she had school the next day. She asked if we could put the top down. I said of course. The weather was very nice. She loves that old car. It is fun to drive. I felt blessed to have it.

I got her home and headed back to our place. I decided to take the ultra-long way home just to enjoy the car and the nice weather. I was thinking it would be a few more weeks before I would be able to drive it again. That chemo was so strong, and I never knew how I was going to feel the next day; round five of chemo was coming quick.

I was just enjoying each little moment I could. I got home and let the puppies run outside. I spent a lot of time walking as much as I could. I was trying to build up some strength and integrity. I was thinking about what the doctors were saying about me going back to work. I felt challenged by some of my doctors telling me that I couldn't go back to my line of work. I kept fighting it and fighting it. However, I was not getting much better.

On top of it all, the next round of chemo was coming. It was another step back. I stayed positive and focused at the light at the end of the tunnel. (My light was not to listen to any negative attitude from anyone.) Over the past week, I could make it down the steps on my own and into the family room and ride the stationary bike. I could only go to a half a mile, but it was a start. I kept pushing and pushing to go further. After riding the bike, I was so light-headed, I would pass out sometimes. I kept the bike close to the wall to rest on it if I had to. And I did a lot!

It was the third week of April, and round five of chemo was Monday morning. I asked Mom or Dad to take me to chemo. Dad had his doctor appointments to get to, so Mom came and took me. We were talking about going to breakfast again. I said that it sounded great. It was nice to see everyone at Dr. Schwartz's office again.

Dr. Melanie said, "Your suite waits for you, sir."

I just smiled and walked with her. She asked me how the exercising was going. I told her about the exercise bike and how I could not seem to get up to a mile without passing out.

She said, "Just keep trying. You are a strong man with determination to survive. It will get better."

I said, "I will keep going, even if it is one-tenth of a mile at a time." I said thank you to her and sat in my chair.

Mom and I started talking about breakfast again. It was sounding good to eat. I reached for my jacket to get out my nausea medication. Just as I was swallowing the pill, Karen was walking by and said, "Did you take your pill?"

I said, "Yes, I did."

Karen came in with the chemo bag and hooked me up. "Your blood work was great this time. Have you been drinking a lot of Gatorade?"

"Yes, I have and a lot of water too."

"That's great."

I said thank you.

"Your weight looks good too."

"I am trying to eat as much as I can."

Really loud she said, "You're doing very good—a lot better than some of my other patients I have!" She said to Mom and I that she was hoping the gentleman in the next room would hear her.

I just smiled at her. I said to Karen, "I feel bad about anyone with cancer but especially bad about the patients that come alone. I pray for them in case they have no one to pray for them."

She smiled at me and said, "That's real nice of you." She left the room.

I said to Mom that a lot of people did not know what it's like to go through cancer, chemo, and radiation. It's a lonely feeling even if you have someone sitting next to you. Just sitting there knowing that you might die at any moment.

Just sitting there, having all these questions and thoughts unanswered, can be enough to be overwhelming with stress. You get the most unsettling feeling, and you cannot wait for it to pass. I just want to say and speak out to you that you are not alone. I do know what you're feeling! It can be scary and confusing. I want to say stay strong and focused on healing and enjoy the rest of your life, no matter how long you have or what doctors say you might have! It helps to say what's on your mind and clear out the unanswered questions, no matter what they are. You have to find the courage inside you to move on and accept your new life with cancer. I did these things I wrote, and it gave me closure and peace in my heart and my mind.

Eight hours of chemo was over, and I felt tired and weak. I said to Mom, "I would like to go home and rest for a while."

So we headed home instead of going to eat. I got home again to a happy greeting at the door by my puppies. I went right to the couch and grabbed my favorite quilt. I curled up on the couch and went to sleep for a while. I woke a few hours later and was thinking about my dream of going back to work. I prayed for a while. I asked God to look out for the people that were alone with cancer and to give them courage to fight this disease. I could hear Leslie's car coming up the driveway.

I yelled out to the puppies, "Mommy's home!"

They all started to bark and get excited. Leslie came in, and we gave each other a big hug and a kiss at the door. The dogs were barking as if they had not seen their mom in days. After that greeting and the puppies finally settling down, Leslie and I talked for a while and decided to go downstairs to watch a movie. I laid on the couch, with Leslie at the other end. After about twenty minutes into the movie, Leslie asked if I was hungry.

I said I was not hungry at all. I paused the movie for her. She went up to get something to snack on. She brought down some chips and dip and sliced cheddar cheese, and some juice to drink. I felt so sick. I did munch on chips a little, but that's all I could seem to eat. After the movie, I went upstairs to rest some more and take my nausea medication. Leslie wanted to watch some of her soaps she recorded. I just went in our bedroom to lie down.

I grabbed the heating pad to warm me up. As I was lying there, I was thinking of a way to help other people that had cancer. I don't have a lot of money, so I could not give any. I was pretty sick to volunteer my time. It was bothering me to come up with a way. An hour passed, and I was still thinking of ideas to help when I came up with this same idea I had months ago: write this book!

I felt if I shared how I got through the stage-four cancers and survived, it just might inspire others to fight for their lives. I have seen so many patients with that "I just don't care" look. They just sat there like zombies, with no expressions whatsoever. When their name was called to go back for chemo, they stood up and walked like a zombie. To me, it felt so good to be alive. I wondered if there was a way to pass on hope and faith in our God and Jesus. This book became a dream and then a reality. I am not a writer, I thought to myself. I was not sure how long it would take to write this, but it was going to happen.

So far, I have spent hundreds of hours putting this book together. Mrs. Sailor, my English teacher who bent over backward to help me, would be proud of me now. I was not the best English student and required more of her time than others. You critics relax on my typos.

Leslie came upstairs and asked if I was okay. I said I was. "I came up with an idea that will not be easy for me, but I will follow through with it." I told Leslie about my idea, and she thought it would be great. She liked what it was about and the idea of helping others. Leslie's an awesome person and gives a lot of her life to help others. After my day, I felt so lucky to have her in my life.

I did okay through the night. I still felt ill, but it was nothing like before. The morning came, and it was back to chemo. I got up to shower and get dressed. Mom and Dad were coming to pick me up to take me. Leslie got up and headed off to work.

I said, "Good-bye and have a good day. I love you."
She smiled and said, "I love you."

I watched her as she pulled away. Dad and Mom came shortly after Leslie left, and we were on our way. They were asking how my night went.

I said, "It was really nice. Leslie and I watched a movie and spent some time together talking. I spend so much time sleeping. I miss her."

Mom asked how I felt.

I said, "I was not as sick as before, but it's more like the flu feeling. The flu feeling was doable to me. "All I can say is you don't know a bad day until they put the nastiest chemo in your body." I feel hungry, if you guys want to go to breakfast."

They both wanted to go.

I said, "Eggs Benedict?"

Mom and Dad said, "Sure!"

Dad said, "We will go, but I am paying."

"Okay, Dad." I just smiled at him.

We got to the Dr. Schwartz oncology office and walked in. I said hello to Penny and signed in.

It was quiet in there today. I was the only patient so far. Melanie called me back and asked how I was doing. I said, "All right. I am going to try and eat this morning after we're done. Enough about me, how are you doing?"

She said she was sad because one of her patients passed away.

I said, "I am sorry to hear that. Is there anything I can do for you?"

She smiled and said, "You are doing it now."

I stood there like a fool for a second and then realized what she meant—be a friend.

She said, "James, can I say something to you?"

I said, "Feel free."

She stared at me eye to eye and said, "You're a remarkable person. I mean, to go through what you have and still have a positive attitude. I have been around you the most, and I have never seen you sad, mad, or upset in any way. You always have a smile on your face and seem happy all the time. I have never seen you shed a tear until today."

I smiled at her. I said, "When you said one of your patients passed, my heart went out to them and their family."

Melanie finished up and then walked with me back to my private suite. I sat in my chair in my room. Karen brought another chair for Mom to sit in. She drew some blood to go get checked. I felt pretty good, so I knew there would not be an issue. I smiled at Mom and Dad and asked if they were comfortable. They said they were. I took my nausea medication. Karen was back quick with the results and was hooking me up. I said, "Thank you. I mean, for everything."

She smiled and said, "I should be thanking you."

I did not say anything to her; I smiled.

Karen said, "I will be back to check on you."

I said okay. I looked over at Mom and Dad and said, "I can't wait to eat. Eggs Benedict sounds great."

Dad and Mom at the same time said, "It sure does."

We talked about politics and the family. Time just flew by. Karen was coming to unhook me. She said she would see me tomorrow.

I smiled at her and gave her the big bear hug and said, "See you then."

I said good-bye to the rest of the staff, and we headed to breakfast. We talked about the family some more. Dad asked how my girls were doing.

I said, "On top, they seem fine. However, underneath, they can't fool the dad!" I took my two fingers to my eyes and then one back at dad. I said, "Dad's watching you," and we both laughed a little. I said, "I think they are doing pretty good, considering the situation. I am very proud of them both."

Dad said, "That's great."

Mom asked about my plans this weekend.

I said, "I am not sure. I don't think we have any plans."

Mom said, "Do you want Outback for dinner?"

I said, "Okay, sounds good to me. I will call Leslie and let her know."

We finished up eating and headed home. I said thank you to them for taking me and for breakfast.

Mom said, "You're welcome. Dad has another appointment tomorrow, so I will come and get you."

I said, "Okay, I will see you then."

The puppies were going crazy as I opened the door. I let them out to run for a while. I decided to hang outside also. It was kind of warm out. I climbed into the recliner and shut my eyes. About an hour later, I woke up and headed into the house. I was feeling pretty sick. I took some nausea medication and went to the couch to rest some more. The phone rang, and it was Leslie calling to see how I was doing. I said I was doing okay, just tired.

She said, "Are you sure you're doing okay? You don't sound it."

"I am okay, babe, just resting."
She asked if I wanted pizza for dinner.
I said, "Okay, but something reasonable."
She said she would handle it.
"Maybe some breadsticks too."
She said okay.
"I love you."
Leslie said, "I love you too, and I will see you soon."

I hung up the phone and lay down for a while. I was feeling pretty tired. I fell asleep, and when I woke up, Leslie was already home and unpacked. She had my pizza and bread on a plate. When I sat up, she was bringing it to me in the living room. She went back to get me a drink and some napkins.

I said, "I could get up, babe."
She said, "I know, but I want to help you."

I said okay and smiled at her. I really felt sick and weak. I forced myself to eat and drink an energy drink. After I ate, I fell back asleep on the couch. Leslie was waking me to go climb into bed at twelve thirty.

I said, "I think I was tired."
She said, "I guess so."

I went in to bed and slept some more. I woke up again about two thirty in the morning. I could not fall back asleep, so I grabbed our laptop and decided to check out the world. I just downloaded Google Earth on to my laptop, and it worked flawlessly.

I went all over the world. I started with Mount Rushmore, and then I went to the Grand Canyon. From there I checked out Hawaii and surrounding areas. I was having a blast with this thing. I went to China to see the Great Wall of China. I checked out Stonehenge and then on to Egypt to look at the pyramids.

I said to Leslie while she was sleeping, "Babe, you've got to see this!"

She said in her sleep, "I'm tired. I'll look at it tomorrow," and she let out a big sigh. She fell back to sleep.

As I was cruising the world on the laptop, the alarm went off for Leslie to get up for work. I said good morning to her. She said, "Are you still on the computer." I said, "Yes, I am. I could not sleep. I was just checking out the Bermuda Triangle area. I was searching for missing planes and ships."

Leslie in a sleepy voice said, "That's nice, honey." She was so cute.

I said, "This Google Earth is awesome."

I looked over at Leslie. She looked so tired. I felt bad for her. I shut down the laptop and got up to go get in the shower. I got out and got dressed. I was telling Leslie how cool the Google Earth program was. I said I couldn't believe the detail it had. I mean, you could count the shingles on our house. I said, "So much for privacy!"

I looked at Leslie. She still looked tired. She said, "I am sorry, I am listening. I am just sleepy."

I said, "Be careful."

She gathered her bags and lunch and headed out. I smiled and said, "Have a good day. I will call you later when chemo is over. I love you!"

She said, "I love you."

"No," I said, "I really love you a lot," and I grabbed her and started kissing her all over her face until she smiled.

After forty kisses or so, she finally smiled and went to get in the car. I stood at the door, waving good-bye to her. She blew me a kiss and drove away. I grabbed my medications and took them along with the nausea pill. Mom came pulling in, and we left for the chemo appointment. I said good morning to her. Mom said good morning back. She looked tired too. I asked if she was okay. She said she was tired.

I said, "Leslie was sleepy this morning too."

We got to Dr. Schwartz's oncology office and walked in. It was super quiet in there again. I hated the silence in the doctors' offices. I said good morning to Penny. She said good morning. Melanie called me back right away. I said good morning to her. We walked back to my suite and got comfortable. Karen hooked me up to the IV. She drew some blood to test and said she would be back. I looked over at Mom and asked if she had ever seen Google Earth. She said no, so I started telling her how cool it was. I told her about all the places I visited. Karen came back with the chemo bag and hooked me up.

I said to her, "How are you today?"

She looked sad still from yesterday. She said, "I am okay."

I said, "One day at a time," and I smiled at her.

She smiled back and leaned forward and gave me a big kiss on my bald head. She turned and walked out. I thought to myself how grateful I was to have people like that in medicine. It takes a very strong person to do what they do daily. God bless them all! I started to tell Mom about how amazing the detail was on Google Earth. She just smiled at me.

So I went on about the Bermuda triangle and how I was looking for ships and planes. I did not find any planes or ships, by the way. However, it sure occupied my mind for a while.

Mom asked if I wanted breakfast today.

I said, "Sure, sounds great. Same place?"

She said, "Yes, that sounds great."

The chemo bags seemed to empty fast today. Karen unhooked me, and I said good-bye to everyone. "I will see you in twenty-one days." We were done and on our way to breakfast.

We got to the restaurant, and they seated us right away. We talked about the family some more and all the drama going on. I felt bad for Mom. She was so nice and sweet and generous, and the list goes on. I did not like the way my sisters-in-law treated her. Mom deserved a lot better after all the great things she has done for them and their families. I just want to say now that Mom and Dad are saints! Maybe you two girls should learn to paddle in your own ponds and appreciate the things you have, like two healthy lungs!

I'm back now; sorry about that! Anyway, we enjoyed our breakfast and headed home. I thanked Mom for taking me to the doctors and for breakfast again. She wouldn't let me pay, okay!

I walked to the door and let those puppies out. It was kind of cool that day, so I went in to lie on the couch to rest. I fell asleep right away. A couple of hours passed, and I woke to Chewie and Ally all snuggled up on the couch with me. Sage was lying on the floor by my head. I felt like we were a pack of puppies. Ally likes to lie across my neck sometimes. Big Chewie likes to be a 75-pound lapdog. I think he still thinks he is a puppy. Chewie has this unique way of opening the door so all three dogs can come in. Those puppers! I kicked everyone off the couch and headed for the restroom.

I came out and took more of the nausea medication and went to lie in my bed for a while. I like playing sudoku puzzles. Leslie had bought me a collection of sudoku puzzle books to play. These helped a lot to take my mind off of things. I played the puzzle game for a while. It felt good that the third day of chemo was over. It was the worst. I was trying everything I could to pass the time and not think about it. I grabbed the laptop to go on Google Earth some more, but the laptop would not turn on.

I used it for five hours straight last night. That must have did it in. I just turned over to sleep some more. A few more hours had passed, and I woke up about 5:00 p.m. I went outside to get some fresh air and walked around the yard for a while, collecting fallen tree limbs. Leslie came home.

I said, "How are you, sweetie? I did try calling you earlier."

"I know, I was so busy today. Did everything go okay?"

"It did, and everything is fine. I was just walking around the yard for exercise. Your nurse friend said hello to you."

Leslie smiled and gave me a big hug and a kiss. "I missed you today."

"I missed you too." I looked into her blue eyes and said, "I love you!"

She looked back at me and said, "I love you so much!"

I said, "What were you thinking for dinner?"

Leslie said, "What do you want?"

A fish sandwich sounded great.

She looked at me confused. "What, no pizza?" she said.

"Fish sounds good."

So we went up to get some local fast-food for dinner. We got back home and headed downstairs to watch some soaps. The puppies were chasing each other around the family room, barking and biting each other's tails. They were funny to watch—just not when you're watching your favorite shows. So I said, "Get down! Shut up!" I got that from somewhere; I cannot remember! It was funny anyway.

It was getting late, and Leslie and I headed up to bed. I stopped by the bathroom to brush my teeth. I went in to bed to lie down.

We were lying in bed, and we started talking about Chewie again and all the crazy things that dog has put us through. The list consisted of one laundry-room door, three dog cages, one garage door, one back door, and the list kept going. He's crazy, but I love that dog. He has separation anxiety. He loves his daddy and wants to be wherever I am. After five years of training, he finally calmed down a little. Leslie and I were at those points with Chewie where we could laugh about it.

We both fell asleep. I woke up about three hours later feeling sick and nauseous. I got up to go into the bathroom. I grabbed the nausea medication on the way.

I sat on the side of the tub for a while. I took the nausea medication and decided to take a shower and get warmed up. I sat there in the tub thinking about the time Leslie and I called to have our carpet cleaned. I asked the woman on the phone to have the people cleaning the carpet call about a half hour before they came. She said she would write that information on the order.

The day came for the cleaning appointment, and the gentleman called as requested. I said to the man on the phone, "I have a black lab that will be outside. He can be a little aggressive when provoked. If you could, just ignore him and come to the front door."

He was like, "Yeah sure, dude, no problem."

I said, "Tell your partner about the dog, okay?"

"Yeah, no problem, dude."

I said, "See you soon."

The guy just hung up. Twenty minutes passed, and they drove up the driveway. The driver got out and started up the sidewalk. The passenger started up the sidewalk and then stopped where Chewie was watching him through the fence. The little Oriental man said, "Look at the puppy. He's harmless. He's just a baby!"

I heard Chewie growl, and I started to go out the back door to say, "Get down! Shut up!"

However, I was too late. Just as I opened the door, I had seen Chewie's backside clearing the fence to go after the Oriental man. I could hear the man screaming for his life as Chewie was chasing him.

"Help me! Help me!" the Oriental man was screaming. "Oh God, help me!"

I ran to the edge of the fence, and just as I got there, Chewie was closing in on the Oriental man. I yelled, "Stop!" Chewie listened and skidded to a complete stop. The Oriental man kept running and screaming like he was getting beat or something. I said, "Come." Chewie came running back to the rear gate where I stood waiting for him. I locked him in the back again.

The other cleaning man stood on the porch saying, "That dude is dumb. I just said to him in the truck, 'Don't mess around with the dog, bro. The owner here has a dog. Did you hear me, dude? Don't mess with him.' Yeah! That was intense."

I just shook my head at the man. About ten minutes passed, and the Oriental man came back. Right away, he started to blame the dog for scaring him half to death. The other cleaning man said, "Dude, the dog didn't do anything to you. You were the dumb idiot who provoked him. Go get the equipment out of the van, dude."

That little Oriental man said, "But the dog jumped the fence."

The other guy said, "Just go get the equipment."

At that moment, I felt like Jackie Gleason in the movie Smokey and the Bandit. I said, "What's the world coming to!" Chewie has never bit anyone. He has chased a couple of people that messed with him. At the time, it was not funny, but now I can laugh about it. Oh, that puppers!

I went back to bed to sleep some more. I woke to the alarm going off for Leslie to go to work. She got up and got ready to go. I decided to get up and watch a little TV. We said our good-byes, and she went off to work.

The three days of chemo were over. It was the beginning of a nice day. I could feel the warmth outside. I decided to have a fire in the patio fire pit. I got out the chair Leslie had bought for me and grabbed the remote to the monster stereo we had in the garage. I was thinking it was time to jam to some tunes. I loaded up the five-disc player with some favorites and cranked it up. I was feeling really sick, but this seemed to help take my mind off of the cancer and chemo. After a while, I let the fire burn down to coals and got up to go for a walk around the block. It was a small block, with just six homes in it. As I was walking, I realized that I was using more energy this way than using the stationary bike, so I kept going. I was taking my time.

Halfway around, I started to get light-headed. I just kept my pace slow! I could hear Chewie whining from a distance because he could not go. I did not have the strength to keep him under control. One thing I had going for me was the five years of saying, "Stop!" That seemed to work with him. I made it back to the patio. Chewie was at the gate to greet me. I rubbed his head and told him he would have to wait for Aunt Kristie to take him for a walk. She came over a few times a week to walk the spoiled boys. I threw on another small log and sat in the chair.

I pushed the recliner out and took a nap; I was so tired. It felt good to get up and walk. It felt like I was getting back a piece of my life, one piece at a time. My brother Mark and his girlfriend, Tara, stopped by that afternoon to visit. They brought the two girls with them. When they climbed out of the van, I said, "How are you babies doing?"

The oldest niece who was five years at the time said, "I am not a baby!"

The little one said, "I'm great, Uncle Jimmy!"

I smiled at my oldest niece until she smiled back. I tried not to tease her but couldn't help myself.

They pulled out some more patio chairs to sit around the patio fire with me. We talked for a while about the family. Mark asked how I was doing. I said, "One minute at a time." I smiled at him. I said, "I have to drink a lot of fluids to keep from getting dehydrated."

He said, "It must be tough."

I said, "It's not that bad," making light of the topic. I just unloaded on him. In a low voice so the rest of the family could not hear me, I said, "It's hard to explain to someone how you feel when your lung was just removed, and it is hard to breathe. Your insides are unsettled.

"My pain level is so intense that I have lost many days and moments with family because I was buzzed out of my mind. My memory has blank areas in it. It's frustrating and a little embarrassing, unless they were in my shoes to experience it. I have lethal diarrhea and migraine headaches. I have to force myself to eat, and when I do eat, everything taste like metal. My ear is ringing so loud, and it irritates the hell out of me. I lost roughly 40 percent of my hearing in my right ear." I smiled and said, "Everything else is going okay."

Mark said, "I am sorry."

I said, "It's not your fault. It's mine. I am the one who did it to myself. I am the one who wanted to be a cowboy and smoke cigarettes."

Mark smiled back. When Mark and I were growing up, we always lived life on the edge. I did not want to miss out on anything. I changed the topic by asking if they wanted to stay for dinner. They decided to pick up some pizza at the local store. We ate and talked about dreams we had and wanted to fulfill. Mark is a country music star. He made his own CD and has enjoyed the music industry a lot. He has played right alongside some of the biggest names in the world. He helped inspire me to fulfill my dreams.

We laughed awhile about a lot of things. One of the funniest things in my family is when we were talking about my mom and how she introduces us to her friends. She says this: "My son, Jim, and this is Jerry. This is my son, Mark. He's a country music star!"

We all laughed a little. No offense, Mom. Anyway, we had a good visit. It was getting late, so they decided to pack up the kids and go home.

I spent most of the next twenty days relaxing outside and having a campfire here and there. I was exercising a lot, going for short walks around the block. About ten days after chemo, my hair started to grow back, and I was not sure what to think. I said to Leslie that I would have to ask the doc what's going on.

It was time for my final round of chemo. I was so excited to get it over with. Leslie was so supportive and inspiring! She was always saying, "Believe!"

Dad had come to pick me up to taking me to chemo. We got there and said hello to Penny. Melanie called us back right away. I said to Melanie, "If Dr. Schwartz is around, I want to talk with him."

She said, "Okay, he is here. Hey, your hair is growing back."

I said, "Yes, it is. That's what I want to talk with him about."

She said she would get him while we did my blood work.

We walked back to the suite. Karen hooked me up to the IV. She drew some blood and said, "I will be right back."

We were waiting in the suite, and I was telling Dad how excited I was for it to be over. He said he understood. He remembered when he was done with chemo. He said, "It's been two months now, and I still have a lot of side-effect problems."

I said, "Like what, Dad?"

"I still have neuropathy issues. I have memory issues."

I stopped him and said, "It feels good to be alive. Right?"

"Right!"

Dr. Schwartz had come walking in with a big smile and said, "How is my miracle patient?"

I smiled at Doc and said, "Doc, I have a quick question. My hair is growing back, and I thought it was strange that it would while I am still doing chemo."

Doc said, "This happens sometimes. Over time, your body becomes immune to the type of chemo you're taking. This happens with most medications. It's okay. I think we're in the clear. Anything else?"

I said, "No, Doc."

He said, "I must go. I have a patient waiting for me."

Dad and I said, "Have a good day, Doc," at the same time.

He walked out. Karen came back and installed the chemo bag. Dad and I were talking about going to breakfast again at the same place. Dad said it sounded good. I was thinking about Dr. Schwartz while Dad was talking about breakfast.

I said to Dad, "I feel so lucky to have Dr. Schwartz as my doctor. I like that he is approachable and easy to talk to. He is very patient and understanding. When I speak to him, it's like he knows personally what you're feeling."

Dad said he liked Dr. Schwartz as well and wished he had him for his doctor while he was going through chemo. Dad said that he liked his confidence and personality. "He is very good at taking care of my son."

I said, "That's for sure." I just smiled at Dad.

Karen came in and set me free for the night. She said, "I will see you in the a.m. hours."

I said okay. She gave me a hug, and she gave Dad a hug too. Finally, chemo was over. We went to eat.

Dad started talking about the chemo side effects and how it affected his memory. I leaned over and grabbed the steering wheel and Dad's arm and said, "You didn't forget how to drive, did you?" I let go of the wheel right away. Dad started laughing really hard, and I began to laugh with him. For some crazy reason, it was funny. We laughed all the way to the restaurant. I was laughing so hard that I started to get very light-headed. I felt as if I was going to pass out. I pulled my seatbelt tight just in case. Dad parked the car, and we sat there for a minute so I could get myself together. We got inside and sat at a table. We ordered up our eggs Benedict and talked some more. Dad was talking about his fishing trip and how much fun they had going.

He said, "It's so beautiful there. You would like it."

"That's really nice, Dad. Maybe someday I will make it up there with you."

I tried to grab the bill when the waitress came back with it, but Dad grabbed it before I could. I said, "It is my turn to buy."

"You buy next time, son."

I said okay.

We walked out to the truck and climbed in. I thanked Dad for taking me to chemo and for breakfast. He said it was his pleasure and thanked me for listening to him. I said, "That's a son's requirement."

He smiled. We got back to my house. I was climbing out of the truck when Dad said Mom would be taking me the last two days. I said okay, and I shut the door to the truck. Dad headed home. My puppies were there to greet me. I let them out and went in the house to rest on the couch.

Leslie came home, and we talked about each other's days. She seemed more interested in my day. I told here about how we laughed about memory loss and forgetting how to drive. Leslie just shook her head. "I guess you had to be there," I said. How was your day, beautiful?"

She began to tell me about her day as we walked out on to the patio. Leslie has a tough career that can be very demanding. She is a social worker for a large nursing home. She is one of those people that I admire for what they do every day. They help the elderly and long-term care patients.

We sat for a while, and I said to her, "I have dreams. One of them is to get back to work."

Leslie smiled and said, "I know you want to make it back."

I said, "If I could make it to my old job, it would be a miracle. I have been writing notes for my book. It's not going to be easy to put together. I can't lose sight of hope and faith. I feel God is listening to you if you give him a chance."

Leslie said, "Those are wonderful dreams." She stood up and said, "Let's get you healthy again first."

I said, "Okay. I am hungry."

She said, "That's why I am going to get you some pizza."

I just smiled. The pizza place is close by, and she was back in ten minutes. We ate dinner out on the patio, and I lit another patio fire. Leslie and I spent the rest of the evening outside and enjoyed each other's company. It was time to take a nice, hot shower and climb in to bed. I seemed to be handling the chemo okay, with a little nausea.

The next morning I got up before Leslie's alarm went off. I went into the shower. I had developed a fever and was not sure if they would give me my treatment today. I took some medication to help with the fever, and after an hour, I was doing better. Mom had come to pick me up, and I said good-bye to Leslie and wished her a good day. She said to be careful, and I said the same to her. I said hi to Mom, and I climbed in the car to go.

She started to tell me about Dad and how he had a fun day. I thought to myself, Thank God. I was worried I disrespected him, talking about the family. I said, "Yes, we had a fun day and laughed a lot. I hope today goes okay." I explained to Mom about my fever, and I was concerned that they would postpone my treatment. It's not like it would be a bad thing. However, I just wanted to get the treatment over with.

We got there and sad hello to Penny. Karen hooked me up and took the blood sample. After that came back positive, we were good to go. I got through chemo, and we went to breakfast at the same restaurant. We ordered the same thing again. We seemed to get the same waitress over and over. She nicknamed us the "Bene twins" on a prior visit for ordering the same thing every time we came there. Breakfast was great, and we headed home.

On the way home, Mom said she would take me to my last treatment. I said okay. I thanked her for taking me. I got home and went into the house to lie down. After a few hours, Leslie came home, and we talked for a while. I said I was missing the old me. I had forgotten what it was like to be healthy.

"That's understandable," Leslie said. "You have an adjustment to make. Nobody likes change, that's for sure."

I said, "I have spent the majority of my life flying by the seat of my pants. I felt that 'spontaneous' was my middle name sometimes. I do not have a problem with change that often. However, this by far was the toughest change I had to overcome." Tonight, I felt defeated again. I felt so sad like never before. I did not say anything to Leslie or anyone else, until now.

As I sat in bed doing a sudoku puzzle, I thought back about my long journey so far and how far I had come since I became sick with cancer. I was still alive and very grateful for that. My eyes started to tear up. I just missed the old me. There is nothing wrong with that, I thought. My heart was telling me I would beat this. It was just one day at a time. I slid down in my covers and wiped my tears on the pillow and went to sleep.

I woke in the middle of the night shaking. I felt so cold. The bed was wet from head to toe again from sweating so bad. I was feeling sick to my stomach and had a fever going again. I grabbed some Tylenol and the nausea medication and swallowed those. I went right into the shower to get warm. After a minute of standing, I slid down in the bathtub and let the hot water run on me for a while. As I said earlier, it helped to think of good thoughts and happy times to take my mind off of the cancer and chemo. I started to think about a time when I first got divorced. I took the girls camping up north in the wilderness. It was Uncle Jerry's place. It was wilderness to them, anyway.

We got up there and set up our large, three-room tent. It was a nice tent that we only used a few times. We put it all together and put our sleeping bags and luggage in there. We brought in the rest of the food and the cooler and zipped up the tent doors. We gathered up some wood and got the campfire ready to go for dinner. I told the girls it would be good to go to visit Uncle Jerry for a little and maybe take a walk and check things out. After the visit and short walk, we were on our way back to the tent.

My youngest daughter said, "What's that black thing on our tent?"

We were pretty far away when she noticed it. As we got closer to the tent, you could see very well. A raccoon was robbing us. That little guy took his nail and cut about a ten-inch hole in our tent and had his front half through the hole. The back half was out of the tent, and he was wagging his tail back and forth like he was the happiest raccoon in the world.

My oldest daughter said, "Dad, what do we do?"

I said, "Stay calm. Let's get some rocks, and we will throw them at him. Maybe it will scare the raccoon away."

So we gathered a large amount of rocks and fired away. My girls did very good at hitting the raccoon enough to where he backed out of the tent.

I said, "It's him or us, girls."

My youngest daughter said, "But look at him, he's so cute. He's probably hungry."

So I said, "I will feed him your dinner then, and you can go without."

She said, "Real funny, Dad."

I tossed another rock at him, just missing him. My oldest daughter hit the coon in the chest with a smaller rock. It was enough to make him run away. We walked up there to assess the damage. He got into the bread and ate half of it. He ate one of the Hershey bars and some of the graham crackers. I thought, Real nice. I got out some duct tape and taped up the hole. I got the fire going and finally calmed down a little.

I said to the girls, "That little guy sure could eat a lot of food."

My daughters were still bothered by it. They both gave me attitude, and my youngest said, "Real funny, Dad."

My oldest daughter said, "Isn't camping fun?"

I said, "Just give it a chance. You'll see!"

It would get better. I was making my famous hobo sandwiches. They were famous for me, anyway. After a late lunch, we hung out with the family. We had some pizza, chicken, and fries for dinner. The girls seemed to get a little more relaxed. By the evening, they were doing pretty good. My brother was laughing about the raccoon and told the girls about the time he had seen bears. That seemed to add some stress to the situation. After a few questions to their uncle about bear sightings, the girls were ready to turn in for the night.

They brought a battery-powered DVD player. They climbed in their sleeping bags and started to watch a movie. Jerry, Ruth, and I hung out at the fire pit talking. After the movie was over, the girls wanted to go to sleep. I told them to zip up their compartment and get some rest. My brother was getting tired too, and we decided to turn in as well. I climbed into my mummy bag and wished the girls sweet dreams.

About ten minutes passed, and my brother yelled, "Lights out," and all the property lights went out. It was definitely dark.

My youngest daughter said, "Dad, can we have a light on?"

I said, "No, go to sleep. Everything is going to be fine."

About an hour and a half later, my oldest daughter screamed so loud! I woke up wondering what the heck was going on. My oldest daughter said, "There's something moving under my pillow."

I scrambled to find the lantern and finally remembered I hung it up at the tent ceiling.

I got the light on and unzipped their compartment. My daughter screamed again that it moved to under her back. I unzipped the door all the way and grabbed her bag with her in it and slid her over to me. I said, "Do you feel anything now?"

She said, "No, why?"

I said, "I want to know if there is something inside your bag or under the tent."

She said, "I still don't feel anything."

I slid her over to my compartment and grabbed my youngest daughter and put her in my compartment. I set the light down on the floor to watch the floor for movement. I grabbed the hard rubber mallet we used to pound the tent stakes in and waited like a man hunting a lion. I had seen the floor of the tent move a little, and I unleashed a good beating to whatever it was with the mallet. I waited a few minutes, and nothing moved.

I said, "There, problem solved. You two just stay there, and Dad will sleep over here." I did not say anything, but I ripped a hole in the floor of the tent. I just put my bag over it and climbed into it.

A couple of hours had passed, and we were all sleeping again when my daughter heard something growl and screamed at the top of her lungs, "It's a bear!"

I don't need to tell you that screaming, "It's a bear," will get people's attention, but I am going to anyway! About thirty seconds passed, and the bright lights came on, and my brother asked if we were okay. I said everything was fine.

My daughter said, "I heard something growl, Uncle Jerry."

He said, "I don't see anything. I will leave the light on for you," and he shut the door.

I thought, Nice. So much for camping. The light my brother left on was so bright that we could have hosted a rock 'n' roll concert. The girls were doing okay now; they both said good night and slept great the rest of the night. The next morning came, and we climbed out of the tent to make some breakfast. I walked over to the fire pit and looked back at the tent. I had seen the hole from the raccoon and started to laugh.

The girls still were freaked out a little and said, "It's not funny, Dad. We are never camping again!"

I said, "Yeah, yeah, yeah, come and eat some breakfast."

It took a couple of years, but I managed to get them to go camping again at a campsite with more family and a new tent, of course. They did not want anything to do with the old tent. I had to go out and buy a heavy-duty, four-season tent with an alarm with motion sensors. (I'm joking about the alarm.) It was worth every penny to get them to go camping again.

As the hot water started to run cold, I stood up. I dried off and got dressed. I was laughing to myself about the camping trip. It helped a lot to take my mind off the situation. I brushed my teeth again to try and get rid of the metal taste. I went to the chair in the living room until Leslie's alarm went off. A few seconds passed, and she asked, "Where are you?"

I said, "I am right here, honey."

She asked what was going on. I told her I woke up with my side of the bed soaked from head to toe and went in and took a hot shower to warm up. I said to Leslie, "Do you remember the girls' first camping trip?" She thought for a second and then started to laugh. I gathered some new sheets for the bed. Leslie helped me change the bedding.

Mom was coming to take me to chemo, and I could not wait to get it over with. Leslie was so excited for me. I was very excited too. I said, "Maybe I can get the port taken out after the test."

Leslie said, "Doc wants you to wait until you pass a couple of tests first."

I just smiled. I seemed to be in better spirits today and focused on getting through this. I guess I needed a good cry. I was not about to feel sorry for myself for too long. That is just not me! I was still alive, and that was good enough. Mom came to get me, and we were on our way.

She was excited for me as well. I said, "I am buying breakfast today."

Mom said, "I don't know. Let's worry about that when you make it back to work."

I said okay. I wanted to treat Mom and Dad to a great dinner and a great vacation for all they did for me. However, it would have to be dinner for now. We arrived at Dr. Schwartz's office and said hello to Penny. I signed in, and Melanie called us back to the suite. I smiled and said good morning to Karen.

She said, "I wish all of my patients were like you. You have such a positive attitude, and I never have seen you sad or depressed yet."

I said thank you to her but did not say anything about last night. She said that she admired my courage through the whole treatment and surgery. She said, "James, you have inspired me and many others around you. Did you know that?"

I said, "No, I did not," at the time.

"I have told your story to a lot of other patients—patients who are in a lot better shape than you were. You are a miracle, that's for sure. I will miss seeing you. You better come and say hi when you're here to see Doc."

I said I would.

She said, "Don't forget about June 8th. Its Cancer Survivors' Day, and the party is at the DMC Huron Valley hospital parking lot. They have ordered a big tent and lots of food. Bring your wife.

I said, "Okay. I will be there."

Mom and I talked a lot about life and how people take it for granted. We talked about politics a little. I said, "It would be nice to see the world with more harmony." I never cared for politics much. I am old-fashioned, I guess. I like respect, honor, trust, and loyalty. I don't like the dirty politics, especially. That just embarrasses our country and its leaders. I personally would love to see a man or woman step up and lead our country with these words and take us to a new level.

I think an untouchable level. America is a wonderful country with many opportunities. I would love to see someone shut our borders down and repair our country first before we help anyone else out. "Once our economy is secure, and our streets are clean from crime, then it would be nice to help our neighbors under our terms. That would be a sight."

Mom just smiled at me. "Maybe you should run for president someday," she said.

"I guess I should." I mean, you never know your destiny. We went on to other topics, talking about food and great places to eat. Time passed quickly. Finally, chemo was over.

The last bag ran empty. Karen came in and unhooked my IV. I stood up and grabbed my shirt. She gave me a big hug and said, "Stay in touch."

I said, "I will see you soon." It was the truth; I had an appointment with Dr. Schwartz the following week.

Mom and I headed to breakfast. We got there, and would you believe it, we got the same waitress again. "Oh," she said in a joking voice, "it's you two again."

I said it in a joking way but with a hint of seriousness, "Careful, waitress! You want a tip, right?" I smiled at her. She sat us down, and we ordered the same thing.

"I will be back," the waitress said. Mom and I started talking about my health and the possibilities of me going back to work.

I said, "That would be awesome someday soon, but there is no way right now. I have been working out and walking. I have a long way to go too, Mom. Only time will tell. I am going on long-term disability this month, and I will be finally getting some income. I can't believe my work would cut my sick-bank funds like that. I feel the funds were misused."

I explained to Mom how I paid into the sick bank for thirteen years. I never used a day. Now that I need it, I got the shaft. "What kind of company could do that to an outstanding employee who has been loyal to them for that many years? I hate greed, Mom. That's what will be this country's downfall." Our topic switched back to politics again. I went on and on about making our country better. Mom just let me vent.

We got home, and I thanked her again for everything. I was tired and needed some rest. I decided to sit outside and enjoy the nice weather. I let the puppies outside and opened the garage to get the recliner patio-chair out. I just loved our little home. It is very peaceful here and has helped tremendously with my recovery. Like I said earlier, the backyard setting is like an up north, natural setting with fallen tree limbs and leaves all over. There is a small clearing in the back where I put a stone fire pit. I used mostly one-foot diameter stones to form the five-foot circle. There are these log stepping pads to walk on all the way out to the fire pit. It's just really pleasant and relaxing.

This is where I spent most of my time when it was warm. I slept in the chair for a few hours and decided to go for a walk around the block. I was thinking how nice it would be to make it back to work. I felt challenged to make it. After a couple of hours, I went back in the house to rest on the couch. I turned the TV on and put on the western channel. I was so tired and weak. I slept for another hour until Leslie came home. The puppies woke me up barking. I yelled "Get Mommy!" The dogs all started barking excitedly and rushed out the door to greet her.

When she came in, she looked so beautiful. She always has a happy smile. I was glad to see her. She asked how my day went. I said, "I am doing okay."

Leslie said, "Do you want to eat?"

I said, "Maybe just a snack tonight.

She asked, "Do you want to watch soaps?"

I said, "Sure, sounds good." So I made my way downstairs to the family room. Leslie brought down a variety of goodies to snack on.

She always keeps my favorites around. Dove chocolates helped a lot with the metal taste from chemo. After a few episodes, I went upstairs to bed. I woke up a few hours later with a fever and totally soaked again. I went into the shower and cleaned myself up. I could not stop thinking about the second-floor wing at the hospital where I had my private room. I am not sure if that was an oncology wing. I am not sure what they call it.

It was always on my mind. There were so many people there with cancer. When I was walking those laps fighting to go home, I had seen little kids and adults there so sick with cancer. Every time, I passed, they were in the same position, like they never moved. I have not seen them walk past my room. My heart went out to them. In fact, I did not see many patients pass my room at all. I said to the therapy person, "Someday I would like to help in some way. I hope to inspire them to fight."

I thought, Maybe I can write something, so they too can understand that they are not alone either and that there is someone else like them. A few times I stopped while I was out walking. I was staring at them, with the therapy person at my side.

She said, "That is so sad."

I just wanted to speak up or yell, "Keep fighting!" At that time, I did not have that energy to share. I told the therapy person how I felt. She smiled, and her eyes filled with tears.

While we were walking back to my room, she said, "I am sure you will do something great for them."

I said, "I will try!"

We finished my laps and went back to my room.

The shower ran cold, and I got out and got dressed. I went to the closet to get new sheets, but Leslie beat me to it. She got up while I was in the shower to change the bedding. She climbed back into bed and went back to sleep. I sat up in bed for a while, working the puzzle book. I was wishing I still had my laptop. I missed it. I liked cruising the world on Google Earth.

The alarm went off, and Leslie got up and went to work. I thought today would be a great day to start walking more. I decided to walk around the block. When I got back from my walk, I went downstairs to the family room and grabbed some one-pound weights. I figured if I was going back to work, I had better push it. So I did.

When I worked out, I was so light-headed and ready to pass out. I lay on the floor for a while until I got some strength back. I went back upstairs to rest on the couch. Later that day, Leslie came home, and we ordered a pizza "again." The pizza came, and after dinner, I went back down to ride the stationary bike. Leslie came down with me to watch TV while I exercised.

Over the next few weeks, I was pushing it to the max, but I could not get over the hump. I seemed to be stuck at a point were I could not get past a half of a mile on the stationary bike. My integrity seemed to be at a standstill as well. I kept at it. I had so much to be grateful for. Sometimes I would look up and say to God, "I need more energy, please!"

THE CANCER SURVIVORS' PARTY

It was June and time for the cancer survivors' party. Leslie and I were going and were dressed for it. It was a Hawaiian-themed party, and I broke out the finest Hawaiian shirt I owned. I liked wearing these from time to time. They seem to bring life to a party. When we got there, the hula girls were dancing, and the food smelled great. We stood in line and were talking with other survivors and staff. Just about all my doctors were there and their nursing staff. It was good to see everyone. We were waiting in line to eat. We approached a table that was full of teddy bears.

This woman named Jan Burlew created a company called Sojourn Bear. "Making cancer bearable" is their saying. The kind volunteer said, "Please take a bear."

I said, "That's okay, thank you."

She said, "Sir, please take one," so I reached for the bear in the back.

I said thank you to her. "How much do I owe you?"

She said, "Nothing. They are free."

I said thank you to her again. They named the bear "Scotty." He was a Scotland-themed bear. He was all dressed up in kilt attire. Leslie asked me why I chose that particular bear.

I said, "Because he is dressed in a kilt with a man purse. He is secure in his bear-hood."

The truth was, I chose him because he seemed to inspire me to smile. He was mine now. I wrapped my lei around his neck and caught up to the food line. I turned back at Leslie and smiled. I put Scotty in her face and said, "Isn't he cute?" She just smiled.

The lady standing in line behind Leslie said, "He is cute."

We got our food and went to sit down. As I was looking for a seat, I was drawn to this table of elderly people. I don't know why, but that's where I was headed. I made room for Leslie and me to sit down together. I said hello to the group of seniors.

Most of them said hi back except for the gentleman in front of me. I looked at his nametag and said, "Hi, Howard!" I just smiled at him. I sat Scotty on the table next to me. I noticed Howard starting to eyeball my bear. He looked at the bear and then back at me. I said, "Handsome little bear, isn't he?" Howard did not say anything; he showed no emotion at all other than the eyeballing. As I ate, I realized I forgot something to drink. I told Leslie I would be right back.

As I stood up, I had seen Howard watching me and looking back at my bear. So I put my two fingers at my eyes and turned my hand and pointed back at Howard and said in a soft voice, "I'm watching you, Howard!" Howard's face lit up, and he finally smiled. He did not say anything, but he smiled from ear to ear. I said, "My bear better be there when I get back." I went and got my water and headed back to the table. My bear was there, and Howard had his smile on still. His wife was smiling at me as well. I smiled back at her.

They had a few guest speakers trying to raise spirits and inspire people to fight harder for their lives. As we all listened, I could not help myself but to watch Howard's expressions. I felt like I was thinking for him. I thought he was thinking, "This guy is clueless on what it's like to have terminal cancer." So I said it out loud so Howard could hear me: "I think this guy is clueless on what it's like to have terminal cancer." He looked back at me and smiled. I smiled back.

I said to Howard, "Even though your days are numbered, try and make the best of what you have left."

His wife just smiled at me. I thought that it was sad that people didn't care enough to fight. I guess we all have a number of days left here. However, my outlook was: why spend them sad and depressed? I told that group my story with cancer as short as I could, and they all seemed to look at me with hope and faith. Leslie and I got up to go mingle. I said good-bye to the group. They all said good-bye back. Except for Howard.

Leslie never said another word to me about it. We walked around the tent and talked with a lot of staff members from the hospital. I ran into Karen from Dr. Schwartz's office and some other staff members. From time to time, I would glance over and see Howard looking at me. I would just smile at him. We walked around and talked some more with other patients and headed home. When I got home, I sat my bear on my dresser where I could see it every day. It makes me think of Cancer Survivor Day, Howard, and that moment every time I see it. I hope Howard's happy, wherever he is.

STAYING FOCUSED

During June, the weather was beautiful, and I spent the majority of my time outside and exercising. My hair was growing in in patches, so I decided to shave it bald again. I started to wash my car by hand and slowly raking and cleaning up the yard. I could not mow the grass all at once. I had a hell of a time starting the lawn mower too. Once I got it running I would mow a few stripes and take a break until I was finished.

I wanted to make it back to work so badly. I pushed walking and exercising a lot. It was not easy, and I passed out a few times pushing it to the max. When I would wake up on the floor or in the chair I thanked God for not letting me die. I can't begin to tell you how grateful I was to wake up. I didn't let this stop me. I was not going to let my cancer be a crutch anymore. I slowly began to work my way up, one tenth of a mile at a time. I finally broke a mile on the stationary bike. The sense of accomplishing this was huge for me! I was so excited and could not wait to tell Leslie. I had kept to myself a lot this month while I was pushing it so hard. I wanted my family to be proud of me and not look at me like I was handicapped. After all I didn't use it for a crutch and I didn't want them too either.

While on the stationary bike I would dream of my bucket list in my mind that I had written. I want to share a few of them with you. I made a long list, and I am currently still working on it.

1. Get my health back the best I can.

2. Make it back to work.

3. Inspire the world. I chose this story to write about. To me, giving is better then receiving in my heart. Inspiring someone to fight for their life is priceless. Watching their faces come back to life with hope and inspiration is incredible. It's truly the best.

4. Be a better dad. Not that I was a bad one. For the record I have always have been there for those babies. I wanted to learn to put myself in their shoes and be more understanding. I guess I forgot what it's like to be a teen or young adult.

5. Get an old motorcycle. Do something that I love.

6. Learn the true meaning of forgiveness and apply it to my life, to everyone.

7. Be a better brother. Not that I am a bad one. I have always answered their calls. I want to try and understand them better to build better relationships with them. We had a rough childhood, and it seemed to put distance between us all.

8. Buy a used corvette if I receive my remission status and drive it year round. Enjoy it until I do not smile anymore.

9. Spend fifteen days in Hawaii. Maybe learn to surf?

10. Travel the USA. I have so much to see.

11. Retire from work somehow and take that time to share with cancer patients. Inspire them to fight for their lives. I would love to go to St. Jude hospital and others like that and share my story someday. Give hope to them.

12. Go on the Ellen show with my story. I think Ellen is awesome and would like my story.

13. Start writing more, because this has been a lot of fun! It also has been a dream of mine since I was young. I was always afraid to write. I was worried about what other people thought.

It's funny how a near death experience finally makes you follow your dreams. Don't wait like I did! Get out there and do it! Anyway, this is my list, and I have had fun with so far. I was determined to make it to two miles.

My breathing was doing a little better. I was still in a lot of pain. My chest and ribs hurt so badly. My back hurt where they cut through my muscles. I was trying not to take any pain medication at all, if I could help it, just at night so I could sleep. Sleep is so important to any recovery.

Leslie and I were talking about getting some work done on the home while it was warm out. I had a lot of work to be done on my home—damage from Chewie, such as door replacements, painting, some deck repairs and fence repairs. Leslie and I went to the local hardware superstore to order doors for the house. It felt good to get out of the house and have some new scenery. I did notice a lot of people staring at me. I said to Leslie, "It must be the bald head, or do I really look like Bruce Willis?"

Leslie smiled and shook her head. She said, "You look better."

I said, "Thank you!"

Anyway, we were getting all kinds of attention while we were out. We chose the doors we wanted and went to the front of the store to check out. I called my brothers on the way home and asked if they could help me replace these doors that were rotted out and chewed up. We set up the door exchange for the following weekend. Leslie and I decided that it was also time to change the garage door Chewie ate through a couple of years ago. Within a few days, the doors were delivered, and I found a great deal on a new garage door. The gentleman came out and replaced it right away. When the gentleman came to install the new door, he was looking at the old door. As he stared at the large hole, he said, "Termites?"

I said, "No, sir, that would be Chewie, my dog! Don't worry, he is locked up."

He finished up and was on his way. The weekend came, and my brothers and I were together again. My youngest daughter came out for the weekend to help paint and clean up.

They got all the new doors installed without too much trouble. Our friend Jill came over to help paint and visit. The weather was beautiful. I lit up a fire in the patio pit and ordered some pizza delivery for everyone. I was so grateful for their help. I was glad to see my youngest daughter. I sat and talked with her while she painted. We laughed a lot about old times when she was younger. She reminded us of the time she was six years old and wanted a larger swing in the backyard. I started laughing at the thought. I began to tell the tale. She started out with this play fort that had a six-foot swing set on it.

She came home from school one day and said, "Dad, we need to talk."

I said, "I am listening."

She said, "Could you make my swing bigger than the school's?"

I sat there a minute and looked out the kitchen door at the fort and said, "I guess so. Yeah, sure I can."

She said, "As tall as you can make it."

I said, "Yes, I can do it, maybe this weekend."

She smiled and went to go play.

The weekend came, and I took her to the school playground to see what I was up against. She pointed out these really tall swings. They measured sixteen feet tall on the measuring tape. I said, "You want them this big?"

She smiled and said, "Yes, just like that."

I said, "I will see what I can do."

We walked back to the car. On the way she had explained that the bigger kids always hogged those swings and she never got to play on them. That was all I needed to hear. Dad was going to hook her up.

We went to the local lumber yard and purchased three twenty-foot 6x6 posts and all the necessary hardware to complete the job. By Sunday afternoon I completed the swing for them to try out. For the record I tested them first. I made this thing as tall as the two-story play fort, approximately seventeen feet tall. When I went to get the girls to try it they stood there looking at it like I had just built Mount Rushmore. They were blown away at the size.

My youngest did not say a word. She ran out to play on it. As she began to swing she yelled, "Thank you, Daddy!" Her smile was so huge and priceless to me. My oldest daughter could not believe her own eyes. She watched as my youngest flew back and forth and finally went out to join her. I said, "Be careful on that thing." I was worried they might get hurt, but I was confident in my craftsmanship. I sat on the grass watching them for hours. They had a blast! They smiled the whole time. Anyway, we all hung out and visited. It was nice to get together with family and friends. I was grateful for their encouragement. It helped me stay focused and kept me on track.

It has been very important for me to find a project or hobby to help take my mind off of being ill. This project alone helped me for weeks. It helped me to stay focused on recovering and living my life! I was not letting cancer be a crutch in my life!

THE CANCER CAME BACK

As the end of June approached, I had an appointment with the radiation doctor, Dr. Hart. Leslie and I went together. We arrived at the hospital and walked into the waiting room. We waited for a while. As we were waiting, Leslie and I were talking about how great things were going. I felt I was feeling pretty good, considering the situation. The nurses had come out and called us back. I went to the nurses' station, and a nurse took my blood pressure and measured my weight. She then took me back to the room where they drew blood.

As I sat in the chair, she was asking me how things were going for me. I was telling her things were going really great and I was feeling well.

She said, "Your attitude is just absolutely outstanding."

I said thank you to her. She was telling me about how inspired other patients were at the party. Some of them had heard about my story. I felt like I did not say much to anyone to have such an impact. I smiled. I was glad to hear that from her. The nurse drew the blood and patched me up and asked me to follow her to the exam room. After a few minutes, Dr. Hart came in, and she had with her the social worker.

Dr. Hart looked really sad and frustrated. So I asked her what was wrong. She said that my picture X-rays from last week did not look very good. And there was a large spot of concern. She said, "James, it looks like your cancer has come back. I am so sorry." She said it looked like it was just underneath my sternum bone and that we need to schedule a bronchoscopy with the pulmonary doctor again. I was looking at the doctor in the eyes; she looked very scared.

I turned to look at the social worker; she too looked very upset. The social worker asked me if I was okay. I just smiled and said, "It's going to be okay, no matter what happens." I smiled. I looked over to my wife, and she already started to cry. I put my arms around her and gave her a big hug and started to sing, "Don't worry about a thing, because every little thing is going to be all right."

Both of them were looking at me as I was singing this to Leslie. I smiled back at them both. I said to Dr. Hart that we will keep fighting. I hugged Leslie some more, and I said, "We just keep fighting and fighting!"

The doctor smiled and said that she would set up the bronchoscopy for as soon as possible. The social worker asked if we were okay. I said I was fine, and the fight was not over yet. I smiled at them and said, "I will see you both in a few weeks, after the bronchoscopy is over. We will go from there." I said thank you to the doctors. Leslie and I grabbed our items and headed for the parking lot.

When we climbed into the car, I looked over at Leslie and said, "Please don't worry. Let's take this one day at a time. We've come so far. I'm not about to give up now. Let's go home, sweetheart."

Leslie was so sad. I kept on smiling at her. I heard what the doctor said, but I was not about to go down that easy. I got home and rode the stationary bike for a little. I walked up and down the steps a little too. I have to admit that I was mad. My fight just was not over yet. Leslie and I ate some dinner and talked for a while.

We sat on the couch and held each other like two young teenagers in love and watched a movie. After all, that was what we were in, an awesome love so special! It is a love that most people search their whole lives for. Every time friends or family are around, they at some point while we're together say, "Get a room, for heaven's sake." It's not like we make a scene. We kiss and hold hands and say, "I love you!" They don't understand we are one now and still on our honeymoon.

As the bronchoscopy surgery approached, I have to admit I was a little scared. I was mostly scared for my wife and my children. I just took things one day at a time. After all, that's all we have anyway. I stayed focused on the positive things in life, like I was still alive. I mean, what's more important than life! I was making progress on the bike and walking. My integrity was getting stronger by the day. My attitude was getting better as well.

The morning of the surgery came fast. It was time to go in for the bronchoscopy. I felt very positive about it. I did not tell the doctor or anyone else that I felt the radiation doctor was wrong. I just knew in my heart that I was okay. Before I went in, I told this to Leslie, and I hoped she believed in me. I was going to prove her wrong. Soon after the bronchoscopy was over, I was awake, and the doctor came in to the room to discuss the results. He was explaining to me that everything came back negative, but there was still a mass there underneath my sternum bone. There was a lot of scar-tissue damage, and it was hard to determine what it actually was.

He could not say either way if I had cancer still or not. He began to tell me of a procedure that's called endoscopy bronchoscopy. The doctor told me that this procedure was very similar to a bronchoscopy, but what they did was cut through my esophagus with a small needle, and it was able to take a sample to test. He gave me referring physician that did this rare procedure. I was very grateful that the doctor who performed this was in my home state. He explained to me that he would be in contact with me. I said thank you to him, and he left the room.

The nurse came and gave me some soda and a muffin. I thought to myself that everything would be okay. I asked the nurse if my wife could come back and that I needed to talk to her right away. The nurse said she would go and get her. I said thank you. Leslie had come back, and I began to explain to her the good news. She had already heard the news from the doctor. He had come out to talk with her right after he was done. I said to Leslie that I felt this was very positive, and everything would be okay. I said, "At least all the tests were negative," and I smiled. After a few minutes, I was feeling pretty good. I got myself dressed, and we were headed home.

The next morning had come, and I got on the phone right away to set up an appointment with the specialist who performs the endoscopy bronchoscopy. The doctor who performs this procedure was located in Novi, Michigan. I was very happy because it was close to my home. The nurse set up my appointment to meet with the new doctor, and it was just a week away. I said to Leslie, "Things are going to be all right. Don't worry. Do you want me to sing to you again?"

She smiled.

As the week went by, I just focused on healing. I spent most of my time outside visiting with my family and friends and burning up some more firewood. The weather was beautiful outside. I was grateful for every day given to me. As I lay in my recliner chair outside, I dreamed of going back to work and getting my life back.

Fourth of July week came, and I was excited to see my friends and watch some fireworks and celebrate our freedom and independence. God bless the soldiers who fight or have fought for our freedom and independence. They deserve so much respect and honor. The lake where we live put together a very nice fireworks display. They launched a giant raft put together by volunteers and launched these huge fireworks. I felt the fireworks display this year was as nice as any display you would see on TV. It's almost as nice as the display seen in Detroit, Michigan.

My appointment with the new pulmonary doctor came quick. I went in to meet him. Dr. Kaplan explained the procedure. He was a nice man and very confident and well-educated. These were the two most important ingredients, in my eyes, for a doctor to have, as I said before. He was very straight-forward about the odds of survival and other issues like my other lung collapsing and death. With my bad luck, I most certainly was listening to him. I explained to the doctor about how glad I was to be alive. I explained to him what I had endured and all of my side-effect issues.

I said that I had lost 40 percent of my hearing in my right ear. I had the ringing in my right ear, called tinnitus. I had neuropathy problems in my hands and my feet. The nerve damage in my feet was painful when I walked. I also had chest pain from the surgery, and where the cut was made, my muscles ached. I said, "That's what I mean by 'bad luck,' Doc. Don't get me wrong. I am very grateful to be alive." I smiled.

Doc said, "Wow, that's a lot. I'm sorry, and I feel bad for you." Doc smiled back and told me not to worry. He set up the procedure within two weeks. He told me I would get the results within two days of the procedure.

I said okay. I said it was very nice to meet him, and I would see him in two weeks.

During the two-week wait, I stayed focused on the positive. I still was not in the clear yet. I visited with family and friends as much as I could. I really did not talk about the up-and-coming procedure with my family. They seemed so stressed and depressed about the news of the cancer coming back. Although the previous bronchoscopy did not show a positive result, my family acted as though it did. They acted as though they were spending their last days with me. I felt sorry for them, and I was the one that was ill. This one day, I sat outside by the fire with some of my sisters, and a couple of my brothers were over.

I smiled at them and said, "Maybe you should appreciate every day given to you. That's what I would do if the shoe were on the other foot. I love you guys! You should try and enjoy your lives. What days you have left. Make each day count as if it was your last. I feel so grateful to have this second chance at life, not that I did not appreciate my life before. I will get through this next procedure with no problems. I can just feel it. I believe! I have faith that God will get me through. I feel that confident."

I smiled at them all. Some of my family members became very distant, as though I died. I would call them. No one would answer. I would leave a message for them to return my call, and they avoided me because I have cancer. I just want to say to them as they read this: I think that you are cowards to treat your own family member this way. I am not only saying this to my family but to any other families who have someone seriously ill. Don't avoid them! They are ill. They need your help!

It was time for the endoscopy broncoscopy, and I was feeling pretty positive. Dr. Kaplan came in to see me just before the procedure. He was very confident and gave me reassurance that everything would be okay. The nurse got me all dressed up for surgery, and away I went. When we came through the doors of the operating room, everyone was ready to go. Dr. Kaplan said in a soft voice, "Any last words, James?"

I said, "Yes, Doc. Could we listen to some Jimmy Hendrix?"

The staff laughed out loud, and the doc said, "That's it?"

I said, "What did you think I was going to say? Beethoven?"

They laughed some more.

The anesthesia doctor said, "Okay, James, count back from five."

I don't remember saying five; I was out. The procedure was over, and Doc had taken a lot of samples and felt very confident that it was just scar tissue. I was relieved to hear it. My wife was so happy to hear the news. I just said, "I told you so, babe," to her in my raspy voice when she came back to see how I was doing in recovery. She helped me sit up and get dressed. I drank my juice and ate some graham crackers. Leslie and I both really liked the new pulmonary doctor.

Being absolutely 100 percent confident helps a lot, like I said before.

Doc asked us to come back in a couple of days for the results. Leslie and I headed home for some dinner. You know it—pizza again!

After a couple days, we were back in Dr. Kaplan's office to get the results. Mom, Dad, and I waited to be called back. Soon, the nurse called us back to the exam room, and we waited for the doctor to come in. Dr. Kaplan came in and told us that he was still waiting for the lab results to come in. He said, "Please wait patiently. I'm sure everything will be okay."

We waited about a half hour, and the doctor came back in with the results. He said, "Like I said, everything came back negative."

He smiled and said, "James, you try and have a good life. I'm sure it's scarring tissue now. I'm sorry about the scare. They probably should have handled that a little better."

I said, "It's okay, Doc. Dr. Hart is awesome and very confident like you. I just knew in my heart that it would be okay." (Having the courage to follow your heart is priceless to me.) I said, "It was very nice to meet you."

Thank you for everything. I shook his hand, and we left the office. Mom and Dad looked so relieved. You could see it in their faces. Right away, I called Leslie and gave her the news. I couldn't help but say, "I told you so," again. We talked for a few more minutes, and then I let her go. I called a few more of my family members to let them know and to help pass the word for me. Mom and Dad took me home. This was a great day for me. I felt now I could put all of my focus on getting healthy. That included eating better.

MAKING IT BACK TO WORK

A few weeks had passed, and I was spending a lot of time focusing on my dream: returning to work. I did away with all of the high fat and high cholesterol foods and began to eat a lot better. Some of the weight I put on soon fell back off as I worked out. Once I got to the desired weight I balanced things off. Who doesn't like biscuits and gravy once in a while? I spent a lot of time on the stationary bike. I was pushing myself to my max. It was slow starting out. My determination and focus was so strong, I was not going to be defeated! Most distance gains were only a one-tenth of a mile at a time, like I said before. Soon, I was up to two miles on the bike. After a few more weeks, I was up to three miles on the stationary bike. I finally was getting closer to my goal I set for myself. It felt so good to set a goal and accomplish it. I just had to spend more time walking and building up my integrity before Dr. L. Schwartz would let me go back to work.

When my butt was sore from riding, I got up to walk and do chores around the house. I was climbing the basement stairs. That helped a lot. My biggest challenge was overcoming the integrity issue where I was getting light-headed and passing out. After a few more weeks of exercising, I was feeling really well. I was near the eight-mile mark on the bike. The light-headed problem was going away, and I felt good to be going back to work, although I did not have the return slip yet. I felt good that I would make it back with no problems.

I finally was up to eight miles on the stationary bike. This was the goal I set for myself. As the odometer clicked over to 8.0 I yelled, "Thank you, God! Yes!" To be completely honest I got up and walked for a while. My butt was so sore, but I made it! I went to the doctors for my next checkup. I was explaining to my family doctor, Dr. L. Schwartz, that I was doing very well. I said I could make it eight miles on the stationary bike. I could stay awake all day now without taking a nap.

Doc said, "You look great! It's absolutely a miracle that you made it this far. So you feel you can make it work?"

I said, "I do, Doc. Please believe in me. I feel everything will be okay."

He said, "All right, I will put your return date for August 30th if you feel you can do it."

I smiled at him and said, "Thank you for everything. If it weren't for you, I wouldn't be here. I can honestly say I owe you more than I'll ever be able to return. If you need anything and I can help, please let me know. This is all I have to offer."

Doc smiled and said, "This is what I do. You don't owe me anything except enjoying your life!"

I smiled back and reached out to shake his hand. We shook hands, and then Doc walked me to the front. Doc looked at me and said, "James, don't overdo it. You're still healing."

I just smiled at him and walked away. As I was walking to my car, I thought to myself, If he only knew how far I pushed it. I got to the car and climbed in. I sat back in the seat and thought back to the day I was diagnosed. I was in the same parking spot, grabbing my phone and making just the opposite call to my wife.

I was so excited. I had tears of joy! I couldn't wait to talk to Leslie! I dialed Leslie's work number. The phone started to ring. The woman at the reception desk answered the phone, and I asked for Leslie. Leslie picked up the line, and with tears in my eyes, I said, "I did it, babe! Doc said it was okay to go back to work."

Leslie was excited for me. She said, "That is awesome. I'm so proud of you. Congratulations!"

I said thank you to her. "I love you so much. I want to thank you for believing in me. You are my everything!" We finished up our call, and I headed over to my boss's office to hand in that return-to-work slip.

On Thursday, August 26th, I walked that slip in and handed it to my boss. The look on his face to me was as if he had seen a ghost. I smiled at him and said, "I will see you on Monday, August 30th."

He said, "Yes, I will see you then."

Monday came, and I was excited to go to work. Once I got there and made it halfway through the night, I realized that all my hard work had paid off. I exceeded their minimum requirements for my return. I know for a fact that all the bike riding and walking I did was one-tenth of a mile at a time, but baby steps can take you a long way. Believing in myself, God, faith, and hope were all big factors in my return. Having those great doctors helped too! Without them, I would not be here. Making it back to work was a big dream for me!

I am so proud of myself! I say, in the end: "If you can dream it, you can do it!"

CONTACT INFORMATION

If you would like to share your thoughts about the book you can do so by going to http://www.miraclejdrstory.com I would love to hear from you. Thank you!

Sincerely,

James D. Richardson